Contemporary Diagnosis and Management of
HIV/AIDS INFECTIONS™

John P. Phair, MD
Professor of Medicine
Northwestern University Medical School
Director, Comprehensive AIDS Center

Robert L. Murphy, MD
Associate Professor of Medicine
Director, HIV Treatment Clinic
Northwestern University Medical School
Chicago, Illinois

Published by Handbooks in Health Care Co.,
a division of Associates in Medical Marketing Co., Inc.,
Newtown, Pennsylvania, USA

International Standard Book Number: 1-884065-18-X

Library of Congress Catalog Card Number: 97-71111

Table of Contents

This book has been prepared and is presented as a service to the medical community. The information provided reflects the knowledge, experience, and personal opinions of John P. Phair, MD, Director, Comprehensive AIDS Center, Northwestern University Medical School, and Robert L. Murphy, MD, Director, HIV Treatment Clinic, Northwestern University Medical School, Chicago, Illinois.

This book is not intended to replace or to be used as a substitute for the complete prescribing information prepared by each manufacturer for each drug. Because of possible variations in drug indications, in dosage information, in newly described toxicities, in drug/drug interactions, and in other items of importance, reference to such complete prescribing information is definitely recommended before any of the drugs discussed are used or prescribed.

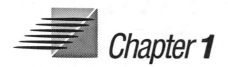

Chapter 1

Introduction

I n 1981, opportunistic infections and a rare neoplasm, Kaposi's sarcoma, were reported in homosexual men and in people who injected drugs.[1] First noted in the late 1970s in these epidemiologically restricted populations, this syndrome was characterized by profound defects in cell-mediated immunity without an obvious cause. Transfusion recipients, persons treated with blood components, women who used IV drugs or had sexual contact with men at risk, and children born to high-risk women soon were identified as having similar immunologic defects and clinical manifestations.[2-4] Before developing infections caused by intracellular pathogens or neoplastic complications, such individuals often had general lymphadenopathy, fever, oropharyngeal thrush, malaise, or diarrhea.[5] Initially, this prodromal illness was termed the AIDS-Related Complex (ARC). The condition was later termed the Acquired Immunodeficiency Syndrome (AIDS). Studies of persons in high-risk populations with and without ARC documented alterations in immunologic status preceding the development of AIDS.

In 1983, the Centers for Disease Control (CDC) developed a surveillance definition of AIDS to track the number of people in the United States with the syndrome. The definition was based on the findings of one or more of the following: specific opportunistic infections that suggest a defect in cell-mediated immunity; Kaposi's sarcoma; non-Hodgkin's lymphoma or central nervous system lymphoma, both usually of the B-cell type; or severe wasting.[6]

In 1984, investigators at the Pasteur Institute isolated a retrovirus from an individual with generalized lymphadenopathy who was from a high-risk group.[7] Within a year, investigators at the National Cancer Institute and the University of California, San Francisco, reported similar findings. By consensus, this virus was named the human immunodeficiency virus (HIV). A second, closely related retrovirus was later isolated from patients in West Africa. The two retroviruses were termed HIV-1 and HIV-2. These agents are similar to a retrovirus isolated from Old World monkeys that produces a clinical syndrome resembling AIDS when inoculated into New World primates. HIV-1 is isolated most frequently in Central and East Africa, the Americas, Europe, Oceania, and Asia. Found in West Africa, HIV-2 is the cause of imported cases of AIDS in Western Europe and the Americas.

Since the initial recognition of patients with this syndrome in New York, San Francisco, and Los Angeles, the disease has been recognized in all the inhabited continents. In fact, infection with HIV-1 has reached pandemic proportions, with the most cases of infection in Africa and Asia. Between 40 million and 100 million people will be infected by the year 2000.[8] The overwhelming majority of infected persons worldwide contract the disease through heterosexual contact with an infected individual.

Initially, in the United States, homosexual/bisexual men accounted for most of the reported cases of AIDS. As the epidemic has evolved in this country, an increasing number of individuals have been infected through use of contaminated needles, heterosexual contact, and vertical transmission. Since the 1985 development of an antibody assay for screening blood, the number of persons infected through receipt of contaminated blood or blood products has decreased dramatically.

Now, 16 years after its recognition, AIDS is the leading cause of death of men 25 to 44 years old and the third leading cause of death of women in the same age group in the United States. It is the leading cause of death in African-American women and of all women of this age group in major metropolitan centers. All racial groups are represented among patients reported to the CDC, although the proportion of cases among white men has decreased. HIV-1 infection has spread unequally into the African-American and Hispanic populations of large metropolitan centers, and among African-Americans in rural areas of the southeastern United States.[9]

Since the isolation of HIV-1 in the mid-1980s, our understanding of the biology of the virus has increased considerably, including its immunopathogenesis, its available therapies, the prophylaxis for the opportunistic infections associated with it, and the treatment of the infectious, neoplastic, metabolic, and neurologic complications associated with it. As of early 1997, however, little progress has been made in developing an effective vaccine to prevent infection.[10] Consequently, there has been a continued dependence on education and behavioral modification to control transmission of HIV-1. Such efforts have resulted in slowing the rate of transmission of HIV-1 among men who have sex with men. In local areas, innovative attempts to reduce spread of the virus among intravenous drug users, such as initiation of needle exchange programs, have reduced new infections among this population; also, antiretroviral therapy has reduced the rate of vertical transmission and the risk of infection caused by accidental, occupational exposure.

The CDC estimates that between 750,000 and 1.5 million citizens of the United States are infected and that 40,000 new infections occur per year, which roughly equals the number of deaths yearly caused by AIDS. Thus, the epidemic appears to have stabilized in this country. New infections occur primarily in young people, especially those living in the inner cities. However, in Africa, Asia, and South America, the rate of new infections continues to increase.

HIV/AIDS is a devastating illness for infected individuals and their families. The pandemic strains the health care system of developed countries and overwhelms those in nonindustrialized societies. The combination of the sociopsychologic effects of the diagnosis, the economic impact on society, and the political-public policy implications of the HIV/AIDS pandemic, all of which increasingly affect marginalized populations, complicates the response to this infection. Much progress has been made in our understanding of the virus, its effects on the host, and its treatment; however, control of this pandemic will require continued basic investigation and augmented public health efforts.

This handbook is designed to provide an easily accessible source of information that helps clinicians who manage patients with HIV/AIDS.

References

1. Gottlieb MS, Schroff R, Schanker HM, et al: *Pneumocystis carinii* pneumonia and mucosal candidiasis in previously healthy homosexual men. Evidence of a new acquired cellular immunodeficiency. *N Engl J Med* 1981;305:1425-1431.

2. Centers for Disease Control: *Pneumocystis carinii* pneumonia among persons with hemophilia A. *MMWR* 1982;31:365-367.

3. Masur H, Michelis MA, Woismer GP, et al: Opportunistic infections in previously healthy women; initial manifestations of a community-acquired cellular immunodeficiency. *Ann Intern Med* 1982;97:533-539.

4. Centers for Disease Control: Unexplained immunodeficiency and opportunistic infections in infants. New York, New Jersey, California. *MMWR* 1982;3:665-667.

5. Abrams DI: AIDS-related conditions. *Clin Immunol Allergy* 1986;6:581-599.

6. Jaffe HW, Bregman DJ, Selick RM: Acquired immunodeficiency syndrome in the United States; the first 1,000 cases. *J Infect Dis* 1983;148:339-345.

7. Barre-Simoussi F, Cherman J-C, Rey F, et al: Isolation of a T-lymphotropic retrovirus from a patient at risk for acquired immunodeficiency syndrome (AIDS). *Science* 1983;220:868-871.

8.   Mann J: AIDS in the world. A global epidemic out of control. Report of the Global AIDS Policy Coalition, Cambridge, 1992.

9.   Centers for Disease Control and Prevention: HIV/AIDS Annual Surveillance Report. 1996;7:1-39.

10. Kahn JO: An AIDS vaccine: Will we have one soon? In: Sande MA, Volberding PA, ed. *The Medical Management of AIDS.* 4th ed. Philadelphia, WB Saunders Co, 1995.

 *Chapter 2*

Pathogenesis
of HIV Infection

Human immunodeficiency virus (HIV-1) replication is an active and dynamic process that begins with acute infection and lasts throughout the entire course of HIV-1 disease. The understanding of HIV-1 pathogenesis has evolved considerably in the past 2 years, primarily because of improvements in the ability to quantitate the number of viral particles in plasma and tissues. Recent studies have clearly shown that while clinical latency may be present for many years, there is no comparable period of viral latency.[1-3] Throughout the course of HIV-1 infection, virtually all infected individuals experience an active viral replication process that is roughly equivalent to the viral clearance rate. Moreover, these patients maintain steady-state levels of virus for variable periods of time. This relationship can be expressed in a mathematical formula (Figure 1). While the typical person infected with HIV-1 may not progress to a symptomatic stage of disease, or to clinical AIDS, for approximately 10 years, the individual variation ranges widely, from 1 to 20 years or more. This variation in disease progression rates can be explained in great part by the steady-state level of total body virus, or set-point, that follows acute infection (Figure 2).

$$cV = N \delta T^*$$

Figure 1: A mathematical formula that shows how viral clearance equals viral production. (c=clearance rate; V=viral load; N=number of virions released per cell; δ=decay rate; T*=actively infected cells. c and δ are relatively constant. Adapted from Perelson.[3]

Phases of Infection

Infection with HIV-1 is characterized by three phases: acute or primary infection, lasting 2 to 12 weeks; clinical latency period, lasting 1 to 20 years; and a symptomatic stage, commonly referred to as AIDS, lasting from a few months to as long as 5 years. During the acute phase following primary infection with HIV-1, viral replication is robust, and measurable plasma viral levels, or viral load, is high. Of acutely infected persons, 20% to 70% are reported to experience nonspecific signs and symptoms such as fever, malaise, generalized lymphadenopathy, and sore throat. A small minority of patients may develop oral candidiasis or aseptic meningitis. Antibody to HIV-1 is typically negative or indeterminate during this phase of infection, while serum p24 antigen and plasma HIV-1 RNA assays are positive. This acute burst of viral replication is followed by a cellular, then humoral immunologic response by the host. Symptoms then abate, viral load decreases, p24 antigen disappears, and anti-HIV-1 antibodies become readily detectable in the blood. The only HIV-1 related physical sign that persists after the acute phase of infection is diffuse lymphadenopathy, which is painless and often goes unnoticed by infected persons.

Following the acute or primary phase of HIV-1 infection, an asymptomatic period begins. During this clinically latent phase of infection, a dynamic viral process occurs, with rep-

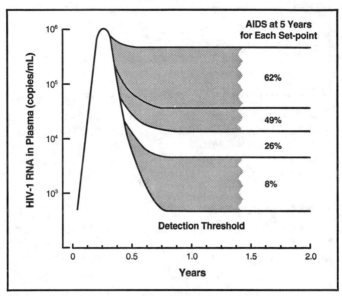

Figure 2: The course of HIV infection. Variable virologic set-points after acute HIV-1 infection and their prognostic value. Adapted from Mellors.[6]

lication occurring primarily in the lymphoid tissue. Using in situ PCR and hybridization to detect HIV-1 DNA and RNA, researchers have found that up to 32% of lymphocytes in lymph nodes have HIV-1 DNA during this asymptomatic period, but most of these cells appear not to be producing new virus.[4] Some researchers have proposed that the continued activation of these HIV-1 infected cells in this large reservoir accounts for the persistent infection and destruction of newly recruited CD4+ cells. It has been proposed that earlier in the infection, the viral load in lymph tissue can be 5 to 10 times higher than that in the peripheral blood. Later in the disease, viral load in blood and lymphoid tissue become roughly equivalent.[5]

Perelson and colleagues recently described observations based on a new mathematical model used to analyze viral

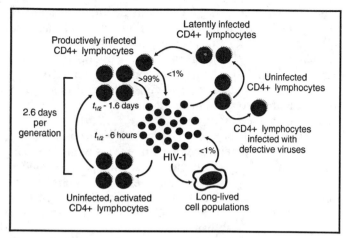

Figure 3: Schematic summary of the dynamics of HIV-1 infection in vivo. Shown in the center is the cell-free virion population that is sampled when the viral load in plasma is measured. Adapted from Perelson.[3]

load data collected from five infected individuals after the administration of ritonavir (Norvir®), a potent inhibitor of HIV-1 protease.[3] In this model, productively infected cells were estimated to have a half-life of 1.6 days and an average life span of 2.2 days. Plasma virions were estimated to have an average life span of 6 hours and an average generation time of 2.6 days; this is the time it takes for a free plasma virion to infect a new cell, which then releases virions into the plasma compartment (Figure 3). The estimated average total HIV-1 production was 10.3×10^9 virions per day, a figure much higher than previously believed.

In these patients, plasma HIV-1 RNA levels dropped rapidly during the first several weeks, following a first-order exponential decrease in viral copy number, with a viral half-life estimated to be 2 days. This decay in free virus particles is actually a measurement of the antiviral effect on virus in the plasma that is a product of the actively producing CD4+ cells.

The actively producing CD4+ cells account for approximately 99% of the total body viral production. The antiviral effect in the lymph tissue is reflected by changes measured in the plasma. The remaining 1% of the virus pool remains in a less well-described compartment consisting of macrophages and infected but inactive CD4+ cells. The cells in this compartment are also thought to have a half-life that has been preliminarily measured to range from 7 to 20 days.

Approximately 30% of the circulating virions and 5% of the CD4+ cells are replaced every day. This figure is a minimum estimate and reflects only those viral particles that are released into the plasma compartment. The number of virions in tissue could be 10 to 100 times higher. Because the steady-state level of measurable virus varies from patient to patient, it is significantly associated with survival and disease progression rates.[6]

With an estimated generation time of 2.6 days, approximately 140 generations of virions are produced over the course of 1 year. The viral pool is estimated to be a minimum of 10×10^9 (10 billion) particles. It is known that only 1 in 1,000 particles is infectious, so that the infectious viral pool is approximately 10×10^6 (10 million) particles. At the reverse transcription stage, errors are made at the rate of 3×10^{-5} per nucleotide per cycle. Considering that the HIV-1 genome consists of approximately 10,000 nucleotides, it is estimated that there is a potential for a mutant variation to occur at every genome position daily. Another way to look at this is that every virion produced is at risk for having at least one mutation. The rapid replication and large population size of HIV-1 in vivo implies that the virus population dynamics are compatible with an ideal Darwinian system.[2,7]

Implications for Treatment

These findings have important implications for treatment and at least partially explain why all attempts at treating HIV-1 with a single agent have had limited, if any, effect. It also helps to explain why combination therapy has been successfully associated with the delay in emergence of resistance to the antiviral agents used. It is difficult for the virus to develop multiple mutations simultaneously, such as is required when combination therapy is employed. The newer potent combinations of antiretroviral agents, which include two nucleoside reverse transcriptase inhibitors plus a protease inhibitor or non-nucleoside reverse transcriptase inhibitor, have been associated with as much as 1,000-fold reductions in measurable virus. In fact, 60% to 90% of patients treated with such combinations have had prolonged periods of undetectable amounts of measurable HIV-1 RNA, even when very sensitive assays were used to detect RNA copy numbers as low as $200/mm^3$.

We must remember that even though 1,000-fold reductions in viral load are now possible, virus is still present during therapy. The possibility of eradicating the total viral pool by prolonged administration of potent antiretroviral combinations is being investigated. While some consider the concept of viral eradication a fantasy, others believe that we now have the tools to test this exciting hypothesis.

Resistance to HIV-1 infection was recently reported in a small cohort of white patients bearing mutant alleles of the CCR-5 chemokine receptor gene. The chemokine receptor CCR-5 was recently found to be a coreceptor essential for HIV-1 to infect target cells. The CCR-5 receptor has been identified as the chief coreceptor for the primary macrophage-tropic HIV-1 strains, which predominate during the asymptomatic phase of the infection and are thought to cause HIV-1 transmission. The mutated gene, which is infrequently found in white but not black or Japanese populations, creates a nonfunctional receptor that does not allow membrane fusion or infection by macrophage and dual-tropic HIV-1 strains. In a study of HIV-1 infected whites, no individuals were homozygous for the mutation, and the frequency of heterozygotes was 35% lower than in the general population, suggesting that heterozygotes may have partial resistance to HIV-1 infection. No one knows whether the resistance afforded the mutation is absolute or relative, or whether resistance will vary based on the mode of transmission. The potential for developing a drug therapy that could block HIV-1 from using CCR-5 as a cofactor is an exciting possibility that will likely be pursued.[8]

References

1.   Ho DD, Neumann AU, Perelson AS, et al: Rapid turnover of plasma virions and CD4 lymphocytes in HIV-1 infection. *Nature* 1995;373:123-126.

2.   Coffin JM: HIV population dynamics in vivo: implications for genetic variation, pathogenesis, and therapy. *Science* 1995;267:483-489.

3.   Perelson AS, Neumann AU, Markowitz M, et al: HIV-1 dynamics in vivo: virion clearance, rate, infected cell life-span, and viral generation time. *Science* 1996;271:1582-1586.

4.   Embretson J, Zupancic M, Ribas JL, et al: Massive covert infection of helper T lymphocytes and macrophages by HIV during the incubation period of AIDS. *Nature* 1993;362:359-362.

5.   Pantaleo G, Graziosi C, Demarest JF, et al: HIV infection is active and progressive in lymphoid tissue during the clinically latent stage of disease. *Nature* 1993;362:355-358.

6.   Mellors JW, Rinaldo CR, Gupta P, et al: Prognosis in HIV-1 infection predicted by the quantity of virus in plasma. *Science* 1996;272:1167-1170.

7.   Wolinsky SM, Korber BT, Neumann AU, et al: Adaptive evolution of human immunodeficiency virus-type 1 during the natural course of infection. *Science* 1996;2:537-542.

8.   Samson M, Libert F, Doranz BJ, et al: Resistance to HIV-1 infection in caucasian individuals bearing mutant alleles of the CCR-5 chemokine receptor gene. *Nature* 1996;382:722-725.

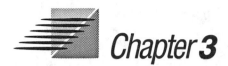

Chapter 3

Natural History

Exposure to HIV-1 through sexual contact, injection of illicit drugs with a contaminated needle, accidental contact with body secretions, or receipt of infected blood or blood products generally results in infection after an incubation period of variable duration.[1] Recently, some at-risk individuals have shown resistance to infection with HIV-1. In one type of resistance, a host's genetic alteration results in the failure to express the coreceptor necessary for HIV-1 to enter cells.[2] This coreceptor, chemokine receptor-5 (CCR-5), interacts with the inflammatory chemokines, RANTES, MIP-1 alpha, and MIP-1 beta. These chemokines have been shown to inhibit HIV-1 infection of cells.[3] HIV-1 must bind to CCR-5 as well as the CD4+ surface molecule to penetrate the target cell. Approximately 1% of whites demonstrate the deletion of CCR-5 and appear to resist infection caused by macrophage nonsyncytium-inducing HIV-1, the phenotype of HIV-1, predominantly transmitted by sexual contact. This deletion has not been found in Africans or Asians, so the documented resistance in these populations must be based on other factors.[2,4,5]

Once the virus has been established, it can be detected in plasma and peripheral blood mononuclear cells by using molecular techniques. Rapidly increasing viral replication ensues over a 2- to 6-week period and is often associated with clinical symptoms. Fever, night sweats, malaise, pharyngitis, a maculopapular rash usually confined to the upper thorax, and generalized lymphadenopathy occur in 20% to 50% of infected individuals. Cell-free viremia can be detected and serologic tests for the core antigen of the virus, p24, are positive during this period of primary infection, which has been termed the *acute viral syndrome* if associated with symptoms. Less common during the acute syndrome are neurologic symptoms, including seventh cervical nerve palsy or aseptic meningitis. A few patients will develop oropharyngeal thrush, sometimes accompanied by esophageal candidiasis. The acute syndrome can last for several days or weeks. We should emphasize that many newly infected persons remain asymptomatic and are unaware that they have been infected with HIV-1.[6]

The differential diagnosis of patients who present with fever, pharyngitis, and lymphadenopathy persisting for 2 weeks or longer includes infection with Epstein-Barr virus or cytomegalovirus infection. A seronegative infectious mononucleosis test should prompt studies to determine if HIV-1 infection has occurred. Some investigators have reported symptomatic primary HIV-1 infection to be associated with a more rapid progression to AIDS.[7] Other studies, however, have failed to confirm this.[8]

With the onset of the immune response, as indicated by the detection of antibodies to HIV-1, the great majority of individuals become asymptomatic.[1] The diagnosis of HIV-1 infection in asymptomatic individuals is usually established by detection of antibody to HIV-1 using an enzyme-linked immunoabsorbent assay (EIA). A positive EIA must be confirmed by a Western blot (WB) assay. The commercially available EIA kits use a core protein of the virus (p24) and an envelope protein (gp41) in differing concentrations to detect antibody. Available EIAs are exquisitely sensitive to detect antibody in 99% of individuals infected with HIV-1 or HIV-2. They are also highly specific; 99% of assays performed with serum obtained from uninfected individuals are

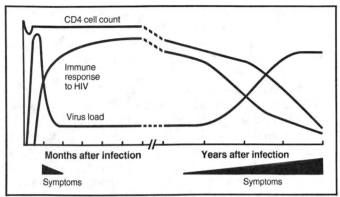

Figure 1: Hypothetical course of HIV infection in adults. (Fischl M. In: *Textbook of AIDS Medicine.* Broder S, Merigan T Jr, Bolognesi D, eds. Baltimore, Williams & Wilkins, 1994.)

negative. Thus, the predictive power of a positive EIA depends on the prevalence of infection in the population. If the prevalence is less than 1%, false-positive reactions can be more frequent than true-positive reactions. Therefore, the confirmatory WB is required to definitively diagnose seropositivity. The WB detects antibody to viral structural proteins and enzymes, bound to a nitrocellulose strip that is incubated with the serum to be tested. The antigen-antibody reactions are seen as bands on the strip. Bands representing two of the three major gene products—core proteins, envelope proteins, or the viral enzymes—are required to interpret the WB as positive.

Individuals in the 2- to 6-week period, before completion of seroconversion, can have a positive EIA, although the WB assay may demonstrate reaction to only one viral protein and be interpreted as indeterminate.[9] Repeat studies 4 to 6 weeks later are usually positive. Some noninfected individuals can have intermittently positive EIA and indeterminate WB assays. Long-term studies of normal blood donors as well as high-risk individuals with such findings have documented that these serologic findings can persist in noninfected individuals.[9,10] The cause of these cross-re-acting antibodies in noninfected persons has not been determined. The prevalence of indeterminate WB reactions among noninfected individuals precludes the use of this assay as a screening technique.

During primary HIV-1 infection, the CD4+ lymphocytes (T-helper cells) decrease,[11] and CD8+ lymphocytes (suppressor, cytotoxic T lymphocytes) may increase.[11] Often, clearing of the viremia is associated with an increase toward the normal values of 750 to 1500/mm^3 in CD4+ lymphocytes (Figure 1). The natural history of the infection from this point on can vary greatly. Approximately 10% of infected homosexual/bisexual men followed in large cohort studies demonstrate a progressive and rapid decrease in the number of circulating CD4+ lymphocytes,[12] which play a central role in the regulation of the immune response. A sustained decrease in these cells to below 500/mm^3 is associated with the occurrence of thrush, hairy leukoplakia, shingles, and bacterial infections. In homosexual/bisexual men, Kaposi's sarcoma can occur when immunosuppression reaches this level. Kaposi's sarcoma is rarely seen in heterosexuals with HIV-1 infection, except in persons infected with a recently detected herpesvirus, termed the Kaposi's sarcoma herpesvirus or herpesvirus 8, that is sexually transmitted.[13] Also, at this level of immunosuppression, persons previously infected with *Mycobacterium tuberculosis* can experience reactivation of their infection. With the continued decrease in CD4+ lymphocytes, opportunistic infections from other intracellular pathogens begin to increase. Pneumonia from *Pneumocystis carinii* is the most common initial serious complication of immunosuppression in the absence of effective prophylaxis, and develops in patients with less than 200/mm^3 T-helper lymphocytes.[14] Individuals with fever or thrush at CD4+ lymphocyte counts above 200/mm^3 also are at increased risk of developing this infection.[15] When CD4+ lymphocyte counts fall below 100/mm^3, fungal infections occur with increasing frequency, usually from invasive candidiasis

Table 1: Opportunistic Diseases

CD4 number	Condition
200 to 500/mm^3	thrush
	Kaposi's sarcoma
	tuberculosis reactivation
	herpes zoster
	bacterial sinusitis/pneumonia
	herpes simplex
100 to 200/mm^3	*Pneumocystis carinii* pneumonia
	all of the above
50 to 100/mm^3	systemic fungal infections
	primary tuberculosis
	cryptosporidiosis
	cerebral toxoplasmosis
	progressive multifocal leuko-encephalopathy
	peripheral neuropathy
	cervical carcinoma
0 to 50/mm^3	cytomegalovirus disease
	disseminated *Mycobacterium avium* complex
	non-Hodgkin's lymphoma
	central nervous system lymphoma
	AIDS dementia complex

and cryptococci, as do primary tuberculosis and protozoal infections, including cryptosporidiosis.

In persons with far-advanced HIV-1 infection, cytomegalovirus, disseminated *Mycobacterium avium* complex infection, non-Hodgkin's lymphoma, central nervous system lymphoma, cervical carcinoma, the AIDS dementia complex, peripheral neuropathy, cerebral toxoplasmosis, progressive multifocal leukoencephalopathy, and severe wasting occur with increasing frequency (Table 1).

In contrast to persons with rapidly progressive HIV-1 infection, approximately 5% of individuals will maintain near normal numbers of CD4+ lymphocytes for 15 or more years.[16] These individuals remain asymptomatic and either have been infected with a less aggressive or "fit" strain of the virus, or are capable of mounting an effective immune response to the infecting HIV-1.[17] The great majority of newly infected individuals, however, will develop progressive immunosuppression over 6 to 8 years. The same HIV-1 related complications seen in rapid progressors occur in patients who experience the more gradual loss of CD4+ lymphocytes. In the absence of intervention, these infected persons develop AIDS and die within 8 to 11 years after onset of HIV-1 infection.

The determinants of the rate of progression of HIV-1 infection appear to be unrelated to race or gender. Older age at the time the patient acquires the infection is associated with more rapid development of clinically significant immunodeficiency.[18] Although the major determinant of the loss of CD4+ lymphocytes appears to be the rate of viral replication, as discussed in Chapter 4, host factors also play a significant role in the natural history of HIV-1 infection. Individuals demonstrating moderate or no loss of CD4+ lymphocytes over 6 to 8 years mount appropriate cytotoxic T-lymphocyte responses.[17] Consistent with the concept of variation in the host response are the findings of an association of multiple combinations of HLA class I and class II alleles, variants of genes for transporter-associated antigen-processing proteins, and a heterozygous presentation of the cell surface chemokine receptor CCR-5 with differing outcomes in infected individuals.[2,4,19]

The clearance from plasma of infectious virions and the decrease in plasma HIV-1 RNA after primary infection do not indicate that a state of viral latency has been induced by the immune response. The virus is sequestered on dendritic cells in the lymphoreticular tissue and continues to replicate.[20] HIV-1 infection, therefore, is characterized by a high level of viral replication during clinical latency and continued destruction of CD4+ lymphocytes, resulting, ultimately, in both profound immunosuppression and concomitant evidence of a high level of immune activation.

Immune activation is manifested by increased serum concentrations of β_2-microglobulin, neopterin, specific cytokines, soluble receptors for cytokines, serum immunoglobulins, and activation of CD8+ lymphocytes.[21,22] Measurement of these markers of immune activation provide prognostic information about HIV-1 infected individuals. Two assays, one serologic and one based on flow cytometry, are especially promising. Tumor necrosis factor alpha receptor II levels can be measured using an EIA. The levels rise and fall in parallel with plasma HIV-1 RNA levels, reflecting the influence of viral replication on the immune system.[22] Activation of CD8+ lymphocytes, as indicated by an increasing proportion of these cells bearing the surface markers DR or CD38, is seen during primary infection and in persons showing progression. In contrast, infected individuals demonstrating long-term immunologic stability, defined as stable CD4+ lymphocyte numbers above 500/mm³ for more than 7 years, show a lower proportion of activated CD8+ lymphocytes.[23] A second, more quantitative approach to the use of activated CD8+ lymphocytes as a marker of immune activation is based on determination of the density of the CD38 marker on the cytotoxic suppressor CD8+ cells, compared to a standard. Studies by Giorgi indicate that stratification of infected individuals according to the intensity of staining for CD38 provides long-term prognostic information early in course of HIV-1 infection.[24]

In summary, patients progress to CD4+ levels of 200/mm³ at highly variable rates. This is the most recent and inclusive surveillance definition of AIDS used by the Centers for Disease Control and Prevention. The replication rate of the retrovirus as influenced by host factors appears to be key in influencing progression. The loss of CD4+ lymphocytes, a state of augmented immune activation, and plasma HIV-1 RNA provide markers delineating differing rates of progression and, therefore, can be used to estimate prognosis.

Once individuals reach an advanced state of immunosuppression, survival remains highly variable. Approximately

40% of persons with less than 200/mm³ CD4⁺ lymphocytes develop within 1 year the opportunistic infections, neoplasms, neurologic complications, or severe wasting that define clinical AIDS, and only 16% of this group of patients survive for 3 years. In contrast, 30% of persons with advanced infection remain free of these complications and all survive 3 years. Clinical characteristics associated with longer survival include maintenance of weight and hemoglobin, documentation of a more gradual decline of CD4⁺ cells to the level of 200/mm³, and stabilization of the count below 200/mm³.[25]

Individuals with far-advanced HIV-1 infection, as documented by CD4⁺ lymphocyte count less than 50/mm³, also demonstrate widely variable survival. Median survival ranges between 15 and 19 months. In one study of homosexual men with less than 50/mm³ CD4⁺ lymphocytes, 30% lived 2 years and 7% survived 4 years.[26] Complications such as lymphoma, disseminated *Mycobacterium avium* complex infection, cytomegalovirus end-organ disease, and *Toxoplasma gondii* cerebritis were associated with decreased survival. Markers of improved survival included African-American race, younger age, higher hemoglobin levels, CD4⁺ lymphocyte counts above 35/mm³, and absence of a major clinical complication of HIV-1 infection despite advanced immunosuppression. Studies of plasma HIV-1 RNA levels in patients with advanced degrees of immunosuppression have revealed that the number of copies per cubic millimeter of plasma HIV-1 RNA can vary greatly. Thus, viral replication may play a central role in determining prognosis in patients with advanced and far-advanced HIV-1 infection. Antiretroviral therapy, prophylaxis for the opportunistic infections, and management of the infectious and neoplastic complications of immunosuppression can alter the natural history of early, progressive, and late-stage disease, which are examined in the later chapters of this handbook.

References

1.   Niu MT, Stein DS, Schnittman SM: Primary human immunodeficiency virus type-1 infection: review of pathogenesis and early treat-

ment intervention in human and clinical retrovirus infection. *J Infect Dis* 1993;168:1490-1501.

2.   Dean M, Carrington M, Winkler G, et al: Genetic restriction of HIV-1 infection and progression to AIDS by a deletion allele of the CKR-5 structural gene. *Science* 1996;273:1856-1862.

3.   Cocchi F. DeVica AL, Garzino-Demo A, et al: Identification of Rantes, MIP-1 a, and MIP-IB as major HIV-suppressive factors produced by CD8+ T-cells. *Science* 1995;270:1811-1815.

4.   Huang Y, Paxton WA, Wolinsky SM, et al: The role of a mutant CCR5 allele in HIV-1 transmission and disease progression. *Nat Med* 1996;2:1240-1243.

5.   Plummer FA, Fowke K, Nagelkerske ND, et al: Evidence of resistance to HIV among continuously exposed prostitutes in Nirobi, Kenya. Abstract WU-A07-3. IX International Conference on AIDS. Berlin, June 1993.

6.   Schacker T, Collier AC, Hughes J, et al: Clinical and epidemiologic features of primary infection. *Ann Intern Med* 1996;125:257-264.

7.   Schechter MT, Craib JP, Le NL, et al: Susceptibility to AIDS progression appears early in HIV infection. *AIDS* 1990;4:185-190.

8.   Phair JP, Jacobson L, Margolick J, et al: Identification of infected persons prior to seroconversion: clinical symptoms and outcome. Abstract 519. 3rd International Conference on Retroviruses and Opportunistic Infection. Washington, DC, January 1996.

9.   Phair JP, Hoover D, Huprikar J, et al: The significance of Western blot assays indeterminate for antibody to HIV in a cohort of homosexual/bisexual men. *J Acquir Immune Defic Syndr* 1992;5:988-992.

10. Jackson JB, MacDonald KL, Cadwell J, et al: Absence of HIV infection in blood donors with indeterminate Western blot tests for antibody to HIV-1. *N Engl J Med* 1990;322:271-222.

11. Detels R, English PA, Giorgi JV, et al: Patterns of CD4+ cell changes after HIV-1 infection indicate the existence of a codeterminant of AIDS. *J Acquir Immune Defic Syndr* 1988;1:390-395.

12. Phair JP, Jacobson L, Detels R, et al: Acquired immune deficiency syndrome occurring within 5 years of infection with human immunodeficiency virus type-1: The Multicenter AIDS Cohort Study. *J Acquir Immune Defic Syndr* 1992;5:490-496

13. Gao SJ, Kingsley L, Hoover DR, et al: Seroconversion to antibodies against Kaposi's sarcoma-associated herpesvirus-related latent nuclear antigens before the development of Kaposi's sarcoma. *N Engl J Med* 1996;335:233-241.

14. Phair JP, Muñoz A, Detels R, et al: The risk of *Pneumocystis carinii* pneumonia among men infected with human immunodeficiency virus type 1. *N Engl J Med* 1990;322:161-165.

15. Kirby AJ, Muñoz A, Detels R, et al: Thrush and fever as a measure of immunocompetence in HIV-1 infected men. *J Acquir Immune Defic Syndr* 1994;7:1242-1249.

16. Muñoz A, Kirby AJ, He YD, et al: Long-term survivors with HIV-1 infections: incubation period and longitudinal patterns of CD4+ lymphocytes. *AIDS Res Hum Retroviruses* 1995;8:496-505.

17. Wolinsky SM, Korber BT, Neumann AO, et al: Adaptive evolution of human immunodeficiency virus type-1 during the natural course of infection. *Science* 1996;272:537-542.

18. Polk BF, Fox F, Brookmeyer R, et al: Predictors of the acquired immunodeficiency syndrome developing in a cohort of seropositive homosexual men. *N Engl J Med* 1987;316:61-66.

19. Kaslow RA, Carrington M, Apple R, et al: Influence of combinations of human major histocompability complex genes on the course of HIV-1 infection. *Nat Med* 1996;2:405-422.

20. Pantaleo G: HIV infection is active and progressive in lymphoid tissue during the clinically latent stage of disease. *Nature* 1993;362:355-358.

21. Fahey J, Taylor J, Detels R, et al: The prognostic value of cellular and serologic markers in infection with human immunodeficiency virus type-1. *N Engl J Med* 1990;322:166-172.

22. Bilello JA, Stellrecht K, Drusano GL, et al: Soluble tumor necrosis factor alpha receptor type II concentration correlates with HIV RNA viral load and decreases in MK-629 treated patients. Abstract 479. 3rd International Conference on Retrovirus and Opportunistic Infections. Washington, DC, January 1996.

23. Giorgi JV, Ho H, Hirji K, and the Multicenter AIDS Cohort Study Group: CD8+ lymphocyte activation at human immunodeficiency virus type-1 seroconversion: development of HLA-DR+ CD38- CD8+ cells is associated with subsequent stable CD4+ cell levels. *J Infect Dis* 1994;170:775-781.

24. Liu Z, Hultin LE, Cumberland WG, et al: Elevated relative fluorescence intensity of CD38 antigen expression on CD8+ T-cells is a marker of poor prognosis in HIV infections. Results of six years of follow-up. *Cytometry* 1996;26:1-7.

25. Hoover DR, Rinaldo C, He Y, et al: Long-term survival without clinical AIDS after CD4+ cell counts fall below 200 x 10 g/L. *AIDS* 1995;9:145-153.

26. Apolonio GE, Hoover DR, He Y, et al: Prognostic factors in human immunodeficiency virus-positive patients with a CD4+ lymphocyte count <50/μL. *J Infect Dis* 1995;171:829-836.

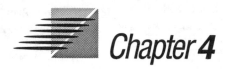

Chapter 4

Measurements of Viral Load

Three commercially available assays can be used to measure the number of copies of HIV-1 RNA in plasma. Only one, the Reverse Transcriptase-Polymerase Chain Reaction (RT-PCR), has been approved by the US Food and Drug Administration. This assay reverse transcribes RNA and amplifies DNA. The Nucleic Acid Sequence Based Amplification (NASBA) enzymatically amplifies the target RNA. Results of both are compared to reference standards. The third assay, the branched DNA assay (bDNA), amplifies the signal attached to captured RNA. All three techniques have little intra-assay variability, and results from each generally correlate well with the others. Moreover, in clinically and immunologically stable individuals, the number of copies remain within a $0.3 \log_{10}$ range. In clinical practice it is important, while following a patient, to use the same assay and the same anticoagulant, and to prepare the plasma in a standardized manner to minimize artefactual variation. In general, plasma should be separated and frozen within 6 hours of collection if the assay is not to be performed immediately.[1-3]

The ability to measure the viral load in plasma has enabled investigators to gain insight into the pathogenesis of

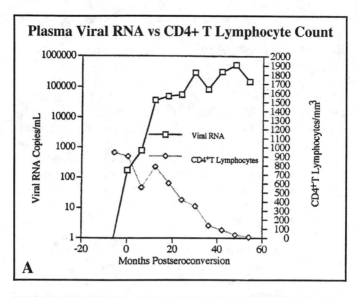

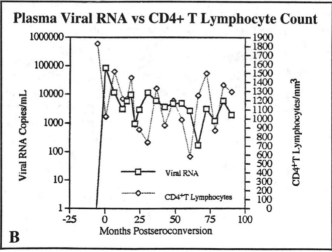

Figure 1A and 1B: Relation of plasma HIV-1 RNA copy number to CD4 in two individuals with incident infection. Zero represents time of seroconversion.

HIV-1 infection, to develop prognostic information, and ultimately, to more intelligently manage antiretroviral therapy. Before techniques were available to measure viral RNA in plasma, clinicians depended on culture of HIV-1 from plasma and determinations of serum levels of the core antigen of the virus, p24, to estimate viral burden.[4,5] Both assays are insensitive. Consistently positive plasma cultures for HIV-1 are present only during the primary infection and in late-stage disease. Serum levels of p24 antigen are detectable during primary infection, before seroconversion, and in approximately 65% of individuals demonstrating progression of the retroviral infection. One third or more of individuals who develop an AIDS-defining condition, however, never have measurable levels of the core antigen.[6] In contrast, cultures of peripheral blood mononuclear cells with current techniques are positive in 99% of all infected individuals. Thus, these assays generally have not been clinically useful. The CD4+ lymphocyte count has been the marker used by clinicians to estimate prognosis and to initiate antiretroviral therapy or prophylaxis to prevent the infectious complications of HIV-1 induced immunosuppression.[7]

Rate of Viral Replication

Ho and Wei used measurements of the number of the copies of HIV-1 RNA in plasma in combination with administration of potent antiretroviral agents (which prevented new infection of cells) to document that viral replication is intense not only during the primary infection, but also throughout the period of clinical stability.[8,9] Figure 1 illustrates two contrasting host responses to HIV-1 infection. In patient A, the number of copies of HIV-1 RNA continues to increase logarithmically and the CD4+ lymphocyte count decreases progressively. In patient B, the number of copies of HIV-1 RNA is maintained at a stable low level and the CD4+ lymphocyte count remains close to normal.

Exogenous events such as intercurrent infection will result in an increase in plasma HIV-1 RNA copy number. With treatment and recovery, levels return to baseline.

Immunization will also transiently increase plasma HIV-1 RNA levels. Other determinants of the rate of viral replication, and thus measurable plasma HIV-1 RNA copy numbers, include the "fitness" of the virus and the host's genetically determined response.[10,11]

When combined with enumeration of CD4+ lymphocytes, the measurement of a single plasma HIV-1 RNA level provides powerful long-term predictive information. Mellors et al documented in the Multicenter AIDS Cohort Study, a prospective investigation of HIV-1 infected homosexual men, that the hazard of progression to AIDS or death over a 9-year period can be established by combining these two values. Among 112 men with <500 HIV-1 RNA copies per cubic millimeter of plasma in 1985, 13.4% progressed to AIDS and 8% died by July 1995. In contrast, of 386 men with >30,000 copies/mm³, 85% progressed to AIDS and 81.4% died within the same period. When stratified by CD4+ lymphocyte number, further predictive information resulted. Only 3.7% of men with <500 copies of HIV-1 RNA and more than 750 CD4+ lymphocytes/mm³ died, while 12.4% with the same undetectable viral load but less than 750 CD4+ lymphocytes died in the 9 years of follow-up. Among the 386 participants with >30,000 copies and a CD4+ lymphocyte count of >750/mm³, 68.5% died; with 351 to 750/mm³ CD4+ cell count, 84.7% died; less than 10% lived 9 years with a 201 to 350/mm³ CD4+ lymphocyte count; and less than 2% lived with <200/mm³ CD4+ lymphocyte count.[12,13] Clearly, combining viral load measurements with the CD4+ lymphocyte count gives physicians important information and helps them determine whether to initiate antiretroviral therapy in an effort to favorably alter the natural history of HIV-1 infection.[14-16]

Saag et al have published preliminary recommendations suggesting that plasma HIV-1 RNA values should be assayed twice before antiretroviral therapy is initiated. Treatment should be started if copy number is greater than 5,000/mm³ and if the CD4+ lymphocyte count is falling, or if the clinical status of the patient is worsening. They recommend that all patients with 30,000 to 50,000 copies receive therapy, regardless of their clinical status or $CD4^+$ lymphocyte count. They suggest that the goal of antiretroviral therapy is to reduce the numbers of copies of HIV-1 RNA to levels that are below the limit of detection or to maintain the level below 5,000 copies per cubic millimeter. A minimally acceptable therapeutic effect is a 0.5 log_{10} decrease in RNA copies below baseline. Clinical trials have demonstrated a significant decrease in disease progression in patients who achieve this degree of reduction in viral load. As therapy begins to lose effectiveness, a return of HIV-1 RNA copy number to within 0.3 log_{10} of pretreatment baseline levels is an indication to alter the antiviral treatment.[17]

It should be recognized that these recommendations are strictly preliminary and based on relatively short-term, 1- to 2-year clinical trials. In general, less potent therapy results in modest decreases in viral load and a more rapid return to baseline levels. Zidovudine (ZDV/AZT/Retrovir®) monotherapy, for example, reduces HIV-1 RNA by less than a log_{10} and levels return to baseline within 6 months. Combinations of nucleoside reverse transcriptase inhibitors, such as ZDV plus didanosine (ddI/Videx®), produce greater, more sustained reductions in viral load and enhanced survival.[18,19] Combinations of a protease inhibitor or non-nucleoside reverse transcriptase inhibitor with two nucleoside reverse transcriptase inhibitors provide the most potent inhibition of viral replication. In one trial, the addition of ritonavir (Norvir®) to ongoing therapy resulted in augmented survival over a 12-month period in association with a sustained reduction in viral load as measured by plasma HIV-1 RNA.[20] A similar antiviral and clinical effect was noted in patients receiving ZDV plus 3TC with the protease inhibitor indinavir (Crixivan®).[21] The combination of nevirapine (Viramune®), a non-nucleoside reverse transcriptase inhibitor, with ZDV plus ddI, was associated with an equivalent antiretroviral response.

The immediate effect of newly initiated antiretroviral therapy can be judged by measuring plasma viral load within

Table 1: Interpretation of Viral Load

HIV-1 RNA Copy Number

Copies/mm^3	Log$_{10}$/mm^3
1,000,000	10^6
100,000	10^5
10,000	10^4
1,000	10^3

Reduction with Antiretroviral Therapy
If Patient has 100,000 copies/mm^3

Log Change	Percent Decrease	Fold Reduction	Copy Number
0.5	66.00	3	33,000
1.0	90.00	10	10,000
1.5	96.80	32	3,200
2.0	99.00	100	1,000
3.0	99.90	1000	100

2 to 4 weeks of starting treatment. However, the maximal response to protease inhibitor therapy may not be observed for 3 to 4 months. Assays should then be repeated at 3- to 4-month intervals to document a sustained decrease in HIV-1 RNA.[13] However, little information is available about reduction of replication of HIV-1 within tissue as a result of therapy. Long-term control of HIV-1 infection will require that nonproductively infected cells, or cells that produce low levels of virions (eg, macrophages and monocytes), be eradicated. The best strategy to achieve long-term remission of the infection has not been delineated. Furthermore, the optimal frequency of measuring viral load in an infected patient has not been definitively established. Information presented at the XI International Conference on AIDS in July 1996 suggested that HIV-1 patients may benefit most by early initiation of antiretroviral therapy and aggressive attempts to re-

duce the level of copies of HIV-1 RNA to below the level of detection. The goal of such an approach is to maximally reduce viral replication to prevent selection of antiretroviral resistant variants.[23] It is most useful to evaluate changes in viral-RNA copies in terms of $\log_{10}$ or "fold reduction." Table 1 provides a means of interpreting plasma HIV-1 RNA data.

Measurement of $CD4^+$ lymphocytes provides additional information to physicians managing HIV-1 infected patients. It is not yet clear that a sustained increase in plasma HIV-1 RNA always precedes a decrease in $CD4^+$ lymphocyte count because the dynamic interplay of viral replication and loss of $CD4^+$ cells over a sustained period of therapy has not been rigorously investigated. Finally, initiation of prophylactic measures to prevent opportunistic infections depends on knowing the level of immunosuppression as indicated by enumeration of $CD4^+$ lymphocytes.[7]

References

1.   Mulder J, McKinney N, Christopherson C, et al: Rapid and simple PCR assay for quantitation of human immunodeficiency virus type-1 RNA in plasma: application to acute retroviral infection. *J Clin Microbiol* 1994;32:292-300.

2.   Kievits T: NASBA isothermal enzymatic in vitro nucleic acid amplification optimized for diagnosis of HIV-1 infection. *J Virol Methods* 1991;35:273-286.

3.   Todd J, Pachl C, While R, et al: Performance characteristics for the quantitation of plasma HIV-1 RNA using branched DNA signal amplification technology. *J Acquir Immune Defic Syndr* 1995;10(S)S35-44.

4.   MacDonell K, Chmiel JS, Poggensee L, et al: Predicting progression to AIDS: combined usefulness of $CD4^+$ lymphocytes counts and p24 antigen. *Am J Med* 1990;89:706-712.

5.   Ho DD, Moudgil T, Alan M: Quantitation of human immunodeficiency virus type-1 in blood of infected persons. *N Engl J Med* 1989;321:1621-1625.

6.   Henrard DR, Wu S, Phillips J, et al: Detection of p24 antigen with and without immune complex dissociation for longitudinal monitoring of human immunodeficiency virus type-1 infection. *J Clin Microbiol* 1995;33:72-75.

7. Stein DS, Korvick JA, Vermund SH: CD4[+] lymphocyte enumeration for prediction of clinical course of human immunodeficiency virus disease. A review. *J Infect Dis* 1992;165:352-363.

8. Ho DD, Neumann AV, Perelson AS, et al: Rapid turnover of plasma virions and CD4 lymphocytes in HIV-1 infection. *Nature* 1995;373:123.

9. Wei X, Gosh BK, Taylor ME, et al: Viral dynamics in HIV-1 infection. *Nature* 1995;373:117-122.

10. Coffin J: HIV population dynamics in vivo: implications for genetic variation pathogenesis and therapy. *Science* 1995;267:483-489.

11. Kaslow RA, Carrington M, Apple R, et al: Influence of combinations of human major histocompatibility complex genes on the course of HIV-1 infection. *Nat Med* 1996;2:405-411.

12. Mellors JW, Rinaldo CR Jr, Gupta P, et al: Prognosis in HIV-1 infection predicted by the quantity of virus in plasma. *Science* 1996;272:1167-1170.

13. Mellors JW, Munoz A, Giorgi JV, et al: Plasma viral load and CD4[+] lymphocytes as prognostic markers of HIV-1 infection. *Ann Intern Med* 1997;126:946-954.

14. O'Brien WA, Hartigan PM, Daar ES, et al: Changes in plasma HIV RNA levels and CD4[+] lymphocyte counts predict both response to antiretroviral therapy and therapeutic failure. *Ann Intern Med* 1997;126:934-945.

15. Paxton WB, Coombs RW, McElrath MJ, et al: Longitudinal analysis of quantitative virologic measures in human immunodeficiency virus-infected subjects with ≥400 CD4 lymphocytes: implications for applying measurements to individual patients. National Institute of Allergy and Infectious Diseases AIDS Vaccine Evaluation Group. *J Infect Dis* 1997;175:247-254.

16. Hughes MD, Johnson VA, Hirsch MS, et al: Monitoring plasma HIV-1 RNA levels in addition to CD4[+] lymphocyte count improves assessment of antiretroviral therapeutic response. ACTG 241 Protocol Virology Substudy Team. *Ann Intern Med* 1997;126:929-938.

17. Saag MS, Holodniy M, Kuritzkes DR, et al: HIV viral load markers in clinical practice. *Nat Med* 1996;2:625-629.

18. Hammer SM, Katzenstein DA, Hughes MD, et al: A trial comparing nucleoside monotherapy with combination therapy in HIV-infected adults with CD4 cell counts from 200 to 500 per cubic millimeter. *N Engl J Med* 1996;335:1081-1090.

19. Katzenstein DA, Hammer SM, Hughes MD, et al: The relation of virologic and immunologic markers to clinical outcomes after nucleoside therapy in HIV-infected adults with 200 to 500 CD4 cells per cubic millimeter. *N Engl J Med* 1996;335:1091-1098.

20. Cameron DW, Heath-Chiozzi M, Kraucik S, et al: Prolongation of life and prevention of AIDS complications in advanced HIV immunodeficiency with ritonavir; update. XI International Conference on AIDS, Vancouver, BC, July 1996. Abstract MoB411.

21. Hammer SM, Squires KE, Hughes MD, et al: A controlled trial of two nucleoside analogues plus indinavir in persons with human immunodeficiency virus infection and CD4 cell counts of 200 per cubic millimeter or less. *N Engl J Med* 1997;337:725-733.

22. Conway B, Montaner JS, Cooper D, et al: Randomized, double-blind one year study of the immunologic and virologic effects of nevirapine, didanosine and zidovudine combinations among antiretroviral naive, AIDS-free patients with CD4 200-600. In: Abstracts of the Third International Congress on Drug Thereapy in HIV Infection. Birmingham, UK, Nov. 3-7, 1996 [abstract OP 7.1].

23. Havlir DV, Richman DD: Viral dynamics of HIV: implications for drug development and therapeutic strategies. *Ann Intern Med* 1996;124:984-994.

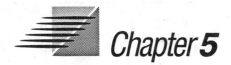

Chapter 5

Antiretroviral Therapy

Exciting and productive advances have occurred in antiretroviral therapy within the last 2 years. Among the most notable advances has been that treatment-related survival was observed, for the first time, in asymptomatic patients with more than 200 CD4+ cells/mm³. Other advances were: (1) a treatment benefit was discovered for postexposure prophylaxis and in acute primary infection; (2) the ability to quantify viral RNA became commercially available; (3) agents in the class of protease and non-nucleoside reverse transcriptase inhibitors were approved along with other nucleosides; and (4) combinations of nucleosides with or without non-nucleosides and protease inhibitors were shown to be superior to monotherapy. These treatment advances were made possible because of a better understanding of HIV-1 pathogenesis, the development and availability of new antiviral therapies, and the ability and ease of newer assays to measure viral load and monitor therapy.

Eleven drugs are now approved with an indication to treat HIV-1 infection (Table 1). These compounds affect different phases of the HIV-1 life cycle by inhibiting one of two different essential viral enzymes, reverse transcriptase and protease (Figure 1). The number of available antiretrovi-

Table 1: Antiretroviral Agents: 1997			
	Nucleoside Analog Reverse Transcriptase Inhibitors	Non-nucleoside Reverse Transcriptase Inhibitors	Protease Inhibitors
Approved	didanosine (ddI)	nevirapine	indinavir
	lamivudine (3TC)	delavirdine	ritonavir
	stavudine (d4T)		saquinavir
	zalcitabine (ddC)		nelfinavir
	zidovudine (ZDV, AZT)		
Experimental	abacavir (1592)	loviride	141W94/ VX-478
	adefovir (nucleotide)	efavirenz (DMP-266) HBY-097	ABT-378

ral agents, including other categories of drugs and those that affect other viral targets such as integrase, will likely increase during the next few years.

Nucleoside Analog Reverse Transcriptase Inhibitors

The nucleoside analog reverse transcriptase inhibitors were the first antiretroviral agents used to treat HIV-1 infection. Five such agents are approved for use: didanosine (ddI/Videx®); lamivudine (3TC/Epivir®); stavudine (d4T/Zerit®); zalcitabine (ddC/Hivid®); and zidovudine (AZT, ZDV/Retrovir®). Table 2 lists the recommended adult dosages and side effects. The first recommendation for antiretroviral therapy was for zidovudine monotherapy. Typically, when this treatment was not tolerated or failed, another nucleoside monotherapy was substituted, such as didanosine

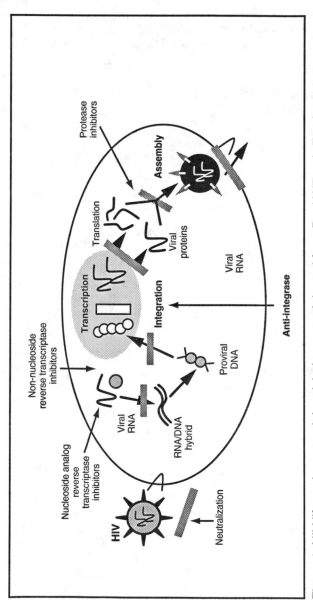

Figure 1: HIV life cycle: potential antiviral targets. Adapted from Paul WE, ed. *Fundamental Immunology*, 3rd edition. Philadelphia, Lippincott-Raven, 1994, p 1386.

Table 2: Reverse Transcriptase Inhibitors: Dosage and Side Effects

Generic Name	Trade Name
Nucleoside analogs	
abacavir (1592U89)	N/A
didanosine (ddI)	Videx® (Bristol-Myers Squibb)
lamivudine (3TC)	Epivir® (Glaxo Wellcome)
stavudine (d4T)	Zerit® (Bristol-Myers Squibb)
zalcitabine (ddC)	Hivid® (Roche)
zidovudine (AZT, ZDV)	Retrovir® (Glaxo Wellcome)
Non-nucleosides	
nevirapine	Viramune® (Roxane/Boehringer Ingelheim)
delavirdine	Rescriptor® (Pharmacia & Upjohn)
loviride	N/A (Janssen)
efavirenz (DMP-266)	Sustiva® (Dupont Merck)

or stavudine. Monotherapy with any antiretroviral agent is generally not recommended except to prevent vertical transmission.[1] This approach, often termed "sequential monotherapy," is now considered obsolete because the antiviral, immunologic, and clinical effects result in a limited benefit that is not sustained relative to what can be achieved with a potent combination regimen.[2,3]

Usual Adult Dosage	Side Effects/Comments
300 mg b.i.d.	abdominal pain, nausea, headache, rash
200 mg b.i.d. 125 mg b.i.d. (<60 kg)	peripheral neuropathy, diarrhea, pancreatitis, must take without food
150 mg b.i.d.	anemia, gastrointestinal upset
40 mg b.i.d. 30 mg b.i.d. (<60 kg)	peripheral neuropathy
0.75 mg t.i.d.	peripheral neuropathy, oral ulcers
300 mg b.i.d.	anemia, leukopenia, gastrointestinal upset, headache, myopathy
200 mg q.d. x 2 weeks, then b.i.d.	rash, elevated LFTs
400 mg t.i.d.	rash
100 mg t.i.d.	rash
600 mg q.d.	dizziness, other CNS

Because of the limitations associated with nucleoside analog reverse transcriptase inhibitor monotherapy, various combinations of these agents were found to be more effective. Four studies have shown a clinical benefit favoring combination therapy: ACTG 175 (asymptomatic adults with more than 200 CD4+ cells/mm³), Delta (adults with less than 350 CD4+ cells/mm³), NuCombo (adults with less than 200

CD4$^+$ cells/mm^3), and ACTG 152 (pediatric). In all of these studies, the only regimens tested were either ZDV and ddI monotherapy or the combinations ZDV/ddI and ZDV/ddC. In ACTG 175, a 45% reduction in mortality was observed with the ZDV/ddI combination and a 49% reduction in the ddI monotherapy arm compared to ZDV monotherapy.[4] In the Delta trial, the mortality reduction was 33% for the ZDV/ddI and 21% for the ZDV/ddC group.[5] In the NuCombo study, it was 12% for the ZDV/ddI arm with the benefit limited to those individuals with little or no prior ZDV use.[6]

In summary, in the large clinical trials using ZDV, ddI, and ddC, the maximal benefit was observed in those patients randomized to the ZDV/ddI combination. The benefits, including survival, were more pronounced in patients with less prior exposure to antiretroviral agents and those with higher CD4$^+$ counts. These studies show that a combination of drugs appears more effective. This is probably because of a variety of factors, including an additive or synergistic antiviral effect, delay in the emergence of resistance, and a decrease in viral fitness.

The newer nucleoside analogs—lamivudine, stavudine, and abacavir (1592U89; experimental)—look even more promising. Although clinical endpoint data are limited, the antiviral effect and durability of the response are much greater with combinations that include these nucleosides.

Lamivudine (3TC) Plus Zidovudine (ZDV)

Four complementary, double-blind, marker endpoint trials were conducted in North America and Europe to evaluate the safety and efficacy of 3TC alone and in combination with ZDV. Commonly referred to as the NUCA and NUCB studies, these studies did not assess clinical endpoints. However, the CD4$^+$ count response and viral load outcomes showed a consistent picture across all studies: responses were clearly superior with the ZDV/3TC combination therapy, compared with ZDV monotherapy or the ZDV/ddC combination. The likely reason for this benefit is that concurrent ZDV/3TC treatment has been shown to delay ZDV resistance, and the mutation at the reverse transcriptase codon 184, Met to Val, that confers 3TC resistance and that rapidly appears during 3TC treatment has been shown to reverse ZDV resistance.[7-11]

Recently, 3TC used in combination with ZDV with or without ddI or ddC was shown to be associated with a delay in disease progression and with improved survival. These results were reported from the recently unblinded CAESAR Study, a 1,840-person trial of treatment-experienced patients with 25 to 250 CD4+ cells/mm^3 (median, 126). Patients in this study had placebo, 3TC, or 3TC plus loviride, a non-nucleoside reverse transcriptase inhibitor, added to the underlying treatment regimen. The disease progression rate for the placebo group was 20%, with 3TC at 9% and with 3TC plus loviride at 9% (P<0.0001 for 3TC versus placebo). A survival benefit was also associated with 3TC use. The death rate with placebo was 6.0%, with 3TC at 2.3%, and with 3TC plus loviride at 3% (P=0.007). Although no benefit against disease progression or death was attributable to loviride, the study was not powered to detect such a difference. This is the first trial to document a clinical survival benefit associated with 3TC used in combination with other nucleosides.[12]

Lamivudine (3TC) Plus Stavudine (d4T)

A commonly used but understudied nucleoside combination is the 3TC plus d4T regimen. One pilot trial was recently completed investigating this regimen. In this open-label and nonrandomized study, treatment with the standard doses of 3TC and d4T was administered to treatment-experienced patients with (1) no prior d4T or 3TC use; (2) prior d4T use; and (3) prior 3TC use. Both drugs were well tolerated and no unexpected adverse reactions occurred. Mean plasma viral load decreases by week 8 were 1.3, 1.5, and 1.0 log$_{10}$ for the three respective groups. The change in CD4+ count was as great as 74 cells/mm^3. The group with the most favorable response was group A, those with no prior exposure to 3TC or d4T.[13] These preliminary results suggest that the combination of standard dosages of 3TC and d4T are well tolerated and effective for up to 8 weeks in treatment-experienced patients with advanced disease.

The ALTIS Study, now complete, was an open-label pilot trial of 3TC and d4T in 83 treatment-naive and experienced subjects with 50-400 CD4+ cells/mm^3 (median=258) and more than 15,000 copies/mm^3 (median=76,502) of plasma HIV-1 RNA. By week 24, the plasma HIV-1 RNA was reduced by 1.66 log$_{10}$ copy number/mm^3, and CD4+ cells increased by 108 cells/mm^3 in the treatment-naive group. In the treatment-experienced group, the plasma HIV-1 RNA decrease at 24 weeks was only 0.5 log$_{10}$ copy number/mm^3, and the CD4+ cell increase was just 46 cells/mm^3. The proportion of patients with undetectable plasma HIV-1 RNA at 24 weeks (<200 copies/mm^3) was 21% in the treatment-naive and 5% in the experienced patients. The regimen was remarkably well tolerated; only one person discontinued therapy because of intolerance to the medications. This study demonstrates that although this is a very potent and well-tolerated nucleoside regimen, it is limited because only a relatively small proportion of patients can reduce their plasma viral burden to undetectable levels. A significantly more potent response was observed among the patients who had been treatment naive at baseline.[14]

Stavudine (d4T) Plus Didanosine (ddI)

The combination of d4T and ddI has been shown to have in vitro synergy and, according to the results of three pilot trials, potent and sustained antiviral and CD4+ count effects. In one dose escalation study, 94 treatment-naive subjects with more than 200 CD4+ cells/mm^3 at entry received one of five dosing regimens of d4T plus ddI. After 52 weeks of therapy, preliminary data demonstrate a mean of 1.1 to 1.8 log$_{10}$ reduction in viral load and changes in CD4+ counts of -22 to 141 across the dosing groups, which favors the high-dose arm in which patients received the standard doses of ddI and d4T. The combination was surprisingly well tolerated, and only one patient developed peripheral neuropathy.[15] The re-

Table 3: Condon Mutations Associated With Resistance in the Reverse Transcriptase Gene

Nucleosides

didanosine (ddI)	65, 69, 74, 135, 184
lamivudine (3TC)	65, 184
stavudine (d4T)	75
zalcitabine (ddC)	65, 69, 75, 184
zidovudine (ZDV, AZT)	41, 67, 70, 215, 219

Non-nucleosides

delavirdine	181, 236
loviride	103, 181
nevirapine	103, 106, 108, 181, 188, 190

References:
Lin PF, et al: *J Infect Dis* 1994;170:1157
Richmond D: *Antimicrob Agents Chemother* 1993;37:1207
Shirasaka T, et al: *Proc Natl Acad Sci USA* 1995;92;2398

sults of this study suggest that the ddI plus d4T combination at standard dosages is quite potent, with a sustained 1-year viral and CD4+ count response. The combination was better tolerated than originally expected.

Two other open-label trials of ddI plus d4T have been undertaken in treatment-experienced patients. Between the two trials, 71 patients who were nucleoside experienced but naive to d4T and ddI received standard dosages of d4T and ddI. After 24 weeks of therapy, CD4+ counts had increased 38 to 50 cells/mm^3, and plasma HIV-1 RNA decreased by 0.7 to 1.1 $\log_{10}$ copies/mm^3. Eight patients discontinued their medication because of side effects, most often peripheral neuropathy. Despite the higher rate of drug intolerance, the antiviral effect observed in these trials suggests that the combination of ddI plus d4T may be more potent than other combination nucleoside regimens in treatment-experienced patients.[16,17]

Summary

Monotherapy with any of the nucleoside reverse transcriptase inhibitors results in a transient immunologic, antiviral, and clinical effect because of the rapid development of resistance and incomplete control of the dynamics of HIV-1 infection. Because of the Darwinian nature of HIV-1 infection, treatment failure is just a matter of time without significant suppression of viral production. The specific mutations associated with nucleoside therapy are outlined in Table 3.

Combinations of nucleosides may delay the emergence of resistant mutants and contribute to improved clinical outcomes; typically, however, these combinations are associated with a more gradual virologic and immunologic deterioration. This is most likely because the synergistic effects of the nucleosides are still not sufficient to suppress viral production in most instances, even though resistance may be delayed. Under optimal treatment conditions, a double-nucleoside regimen would be expected to reduce plasma viral burden to below detectable levels (<200 copies/mm^3) in up to 20% of instances, regardless of the regimen chosen.

The best use for nucleoside reverse transcriptase inhibitors is in combination with other antiretroviral agents of different classes, such as the non-nucleosides or protease inhibitors. When choosing a combination, clinicians must consider synergy, resistance profile, and toxicities. Table 4 outlines the various combinations that have been studied. Note that the degree of study varies tremendously between the regimens, primarily because of the time of development and manufacturer. For example, didanosine (ddI) plus zidovudine (ZDV) is the most studied combination and has been tested in thousands of patients. However, the most potent combination is most likely 3TC plus stavudine (d4T). This combination also is the best tolerated and a popular choice despite the fact that data exist on 116 patients studied prospectively.

The decision to use a particular nucleoside combination should be based on available clinical data about the combina-

Table 4: Nucleoside Reverse Transcriptase Inhibitor Combinations

zidovudine + didanosine	most studied combination; survival enhanced compared with zidovudine monotherapy or zidovudine plus zalcitabine
zidovudine + zalcitabine	well-studied combination; not as effective as zidovudine plus didanosine, but more effective than zidovudine monotherapy in treatment-naive patients
zidovudine + lamivudine	more potent and sustained antiviral/immunologic effect compared to zidovudine monotherapy or to a combination with didanosine or zalcitabine
didanosine + stavudine	potent and sustained antiviral/immunologic effect compared with other nucleoside combinations; studied in only 165 patients to date, all with more than 200 CD4 cells/mm^3; peripheral neuropathy noted in fewer patients than expected
stavudine + lamivudine	prospectively studied in fewer than 116 patients; those with no prior exposure to either agent did best; well tolerated
didanosine + zalcitabine	not recommended because of overlapping toxicity of peripheral neuropathy
stavudine + zidovudine	these thymidine analogs are not recommended in combination because of antagonism and enhanced cellular toxicity when used together
didanosine + 3TC	not recommended because of potential antagonism
zalcitabine + 3TC	no information available
triple nucleoside combinations	limited information available

	Dose	Side Effects
delavirdine	400 mg t.i.d.	rash 35%
loviride	100 mg t.i.d.	rash 5% diarrhea 11%
nevirapine	200 mg q.d. x 2 wks then 200 mg b.i.d.	rash 17%
efavirenz (not pictured)	600 mg q.d.	dizziness 5% - 10%

Figure 2: Non-nucleoside reverse transcriptase inhibitors: dosage and side effects.

tion being considered, tolerability of the agents, acceptance by the patient, and prior nucleoside use, if any (Table 4).

Non-Nucleoside Reverse Transcriptase Inhibitor Therapy

The non-nucleoside reverse transcriptase inhibitors are a structurally diverse group of compounds with functional similarities (Figure 2). These agents have been developed by several pharmaceutical firms because of their ability to inhibit HIV-1 reverse transcriptase. As a result, these compounds have been shown to inhibit HIV-1 reverse transcriptase, but not that of HIV-2 or other retrovirus enzymes, nor do they inhibit any human enzymatic systems. In general, these molecules are small, relatively easy to manufacture, can be widely and rapidly disseminated into body tissues, and exhibit a nonoverlapping toxicity profile compared with other antiretroviral agents.[18] The dosages and side effects of the four most studied non-nucleosides are listed in Figure 2.

The mode of action of the non-nucleosides is direct reverse transcriptase inhibition. No intracellular metabolism of these agents is required. The site of action within the reverse transcriptase enzyme is distinct from the catalytic site. Unlike the nucleosides, chain termination of the transcribed RNA does not occur. The inhibition of the enzyme depends on this process.[19,20]

The clinical history of non-nucleoside reverse transcriptase inhibitors has been checkered. Originally, the combination of nevirapine (Viramune®), the prototype non-nucleoside, with didanosine plus zidovudine appeared to result in *convergence* and complete termination of viral replication in vitro. Although this turned out not to be the case, clinical development continued. Early studies, demonstrating marginal benefits in treatment-experienced patients, were not encouraging. However, treatment in combination with at least two other agents, both nucleosides, in patients without prior therapy resulted in surprising antiviral and immunologic benefit, as described below.

Nevirapine

Early studies with nevirapine involved patients with relatively advanced disease and significant prior exposure to zidovudine. Nevertheless, nevirapine therapy was associated with an improved, although not dramatic, reduction in viral load and increase in $CD4^+$ cell count when compared with continuing therapy with zidovudine, didanosine, or the combination of both. More recent investigations demonstrated dramatic increases in $CD4^+$ counts and decreases in viral load when nevirapine was used in combination with two nucleosides in patients who had been antiretroviral treatment naive.[21]

Nevirapine is a chemically synthesized small molecule that is a non-nucleoside inhibitor of HIV-1 reverse transcriptase. It is commercially available in a 200-mg tablet, but has been made into a suspension, a solution, and intravenous injection for use in clinical trials. Nevirapine is selective for HIV-1 reverse transcriptase and has no known effect on other cellular enzymes, such as human DNA polymerases, calf thymus DNA polymerases, and human plasma renin. Nevirapine has no observable cytotoxic effect on cells in general.

Overall, the pharmacokinetics of nevirapine are characterized by rapid and nearly complete oral absorption, an apparent volume of distribution that exceeds total body water, and a prolonged disposition phase in humans. Metabolic autoinduction of cytochrome P-450 isoenzymes results in a 1.5- to 2.0-fold increase in nevirapine systemic clearance after 1 to 2 weeks of administration. This in turn results in a terminal phase half-life of 25 to 30 hours after multiple dosings. Because of this phenomenon, the recommended adult dosage is 200 mg daily for the first 2 weeks, then 200 mg given twice daily.

Nevirapine penetrates all tissues, including human cerebral spinal fluid where levels are approximately equal to the plasma fraction not bound to protein (45%). There are no known significant drug interactions. However, concomitant use with protease inhibitors may result in significant changes in the rate of metabolism of the protease inhibitor. The metabolic rate may either increase or decrease, depending on the specific non-nucleoside. When nevirapine was used in two- and three-drug combinations with nucleoside analogs, the antiviral activity was usually synergistic or at least additive in vitro.[22-24]

The resistance profile of nevirapine overlaps with the other non-nucleoside reverse transcriptase inhibitors, but not with nucleosides or protease inhibitors (Table 3). In clinical studies, reduced sensitivity to nevirapine can be attributed to the presence of mutations within the binding pocket on reverse transcriptase. During monotherapy with nevirapine, emergence of resistance is rapid, with amino acid changes predominantly seen at position 181 and, to a lesser extent, at sites 103, 106, 108, 188, and 190. When used in combina-

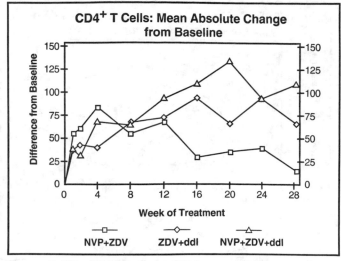

Figure 3: The INCAS study: CD4+ count responses in each group over the first 28 weeks.

tion, the 181 mutation is less frequent and the resistance pattern is different.[25]

Nevirapine was approved based on surrogate marker endpoint studies from five clinical trials. Three of the more relevant studies are discussed below.

The INCAS Study

The most impressive data to date about the non-nucleosides are from the INCAS Study, a 151-patient trial in treatment-naive persons with 200 to 600 CD4+ cells/mm³ (mean, 376). The treatment arms included standard doses of ZDV administered with nevirapine, ddI, or both. The surprising interim results, as shown in Figures 3, 4, and 5, demonstrated that the nevirapine/ddI/ZDV group had the highest rise in CD4+ cell count (120 cells/mm³), the greatest decrease in HIV-1 RNA from baseline (1.7 $\log_{10}$), and the greatest proportion of patients with undetectable virus after 52 weeks (67%), which was clearly superior to the groups

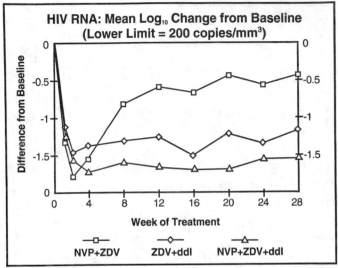

Figure 4: The INCAS study: Viral RNA response in each treatment group.

treated with nevirapine/ZDV and ddI/ZDV.[26] These results suggest that nevirapine given with two nucleosides is a potent therapeutic regimen in patients with mild to moderately advanced HIV-1 disease and no history of prior antiretroviral treatment.

Nevirapine Plus Didanosine and Zidovudine: ACTG 241

The largest complete comparative trial involved 398 patients with $CD4^+$ counts <350 cells/mm^3 (median, 138) and a history of prior nucleoside experience (median, 115 weeks). Patients were randomized to receive nevirapine + ddI + ZDV or the nucleoside combination ddI + ZDV. The nevirapine-containing group had a maximum increase from baseline in $CD4^+$ count of 34 cells/mm^3 versus 11.3 cells for the nucleoside-only group. The mean value for $CD4^+$ cells remained above baseline for the nevirapine-containing group throughout the 48-week period, compared to only 24 weeks for the

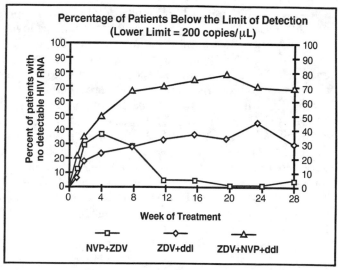

Figure 5: The INCAS study: Population of patients with undetectable viral load.

nucleoside-only arm. The maximum decrease in HIV-1 RNA from baseline was 1.16 log copies/mm³, which remained below baseline for 48 weeks in the nevirapine-containing arm versus 0.45 $\log_{10}$ copies/mm³ for the nucleoside-only group, which returned to baseline after 32 weeks. The patients with the best response were those who had received only zidovudine in the past and those with more than 200 CD4⁺ cells/mm³ at baseline. There were no differences in clinical endpoints (this was not powered as a clinical endpoint trial).[27]

Nevirapine Plus Didanosine and Zidovudine: ACTG 193a

The ACTG 193a study involved 1,313 patients with significantly advanced disease. All subjects had less than 50 CD4⁺ cells/mm³ (mean, 20) and 82% had received therapy with nucleoside analogs before entering the study. Eligible patients received one of four regimens; all drugs were administered in standard dosages: (1) ZDV alternating with ddI; (2) ZDV plus ddC; (3) ZDV plus ddI; or (4) nevirapine and ddI plus ZDV. The triple-therapy group had the lowest mortality rate (36%) and the longest survival rate (112 weeks). Patients receiving the triple-therapy regimen experienced a statistically significant benefit, compared to the other treatment arms. Pairwise comparisons were significant only for the triple-therapy group, compared with groups 1 and 2. No statistically significant difference existed between the nevirapine/ddI/ZDV and ddI/ZDV treatment groups. However, an analysis of patients who received study drugs and who were treatment experienced (82%) yielded a significant difference (P=0.02) between the two treatment arms.

This trial was plagued by a high mortality rate and intolerance to all the treatment regimens, although there was no difference in the number of adverse events between study arms. Seventy-four percent of subjects were not on assigned medication at the end of the trial or at the time of death.[28,29] The results from this study suggest a favorable, albeit modest, clinical benefit associated with a triple-drug, nevirapine-containing regimen for patients with advanced AIDS.

Safety/Tolerability

With the exception of rash, no significantly higher rates of adverse events have been documented in nevirapine-treated patients compared to non-nevirapine groups treated in the comparative trials. Most of these rashes are nonspecific, maculopapular, and mild to moderate in severity. In general, the rashes are self-limited, occur within the first month of therapy, and require drug discontinuation in only about 6% of cases. The incidence of Stevens-Johnson syndrome across all trials is 0.5% (8/1,752 patients); none of these cases resulted in a fatality. Liver transaminase level elevations have been observed during nevirapine therapy.

Delavirdine

Delavirdine (Rescriptor®) is the second non-nucleoside reverse transcriptase inhibitor approved. Although delavirdine has been extensively studied in more than 2,700 patients, little data have actually been published about its efficacy.

Although in many ways similar to nevirapine, delavirdine is different in that it must be dosed three times daily and it does not significantly cross the blood-brain barrier. Resistance is overlapping with that of the non-nucleoside reverse transcriptase inhibitors, and its main side effect, rash, is similar to that observed with nevirapine therapy.

Preliminary results from two large studies in 1,700 patients have been made partially available. In Protocol 017, treatment-experienced patients with less than 300 CD4+ cells/mm^3 (mean, 135) were randomized to receive delavirdine 400 mg 3 times daily plus ddI or ddI alone. In Protocol 021, patients with 200 to 500 CD4+ cells/mm^3 (mean, 325) were randomized to receive ZDV plus delavirdine at 200 mg, 300 mg, or 400 mg 3 times daily.[25] After a 6-month planned interim analysis, the Protocol 017 trial was stopped after it found that there was no statistical difference between the ddI and the ddI + delavirdine arms regarding death or disease progression. In Protocol 021, which involved a group of patients with much less prior treatment, subjects who received delavirdine 300 or 400 mg 3 times daily did marginally better than those who were randomized to receive zidovudine alone or in combination with lower delavirdine doses.[30-32] Exactly what population is likely to benefit from a treatment regimen that includes delavirdine remains to be determined.

Loviride

Loviride, another non-nucleoside being studied, has been shown to have an antiviral and CD4+ cell count effect in HIV-1 infected patients.[33] Two completed pivotal trials assessed the potential for the use of loviride.

Nucleoside Therapy Plus 3TC or 3TC Plus Loviride: The CAESAR Study

CAESAR was an international study that enrolled 1,892 subjects with CD4+ cell counts between 25 and 250/mm^3. Patients were randomized to add to their nucleoside regimen placebo, 3TC, or the combination 3TC/loviride. The rate of disease progression or death was 20% in the placebo group, versus 9% for those adding 3TC or 3TC/loviride. Mortality alone also was lower in the regimens that contained 3TC ($P=0.0007$). There was no statistical difference in clinical endpoints or mortality for patients adding 3TC, versus those adding 3TC/loviride. No clear-cut advantage was observed for the cohort that added loviride to the regimen.

AZT/3TC Plus Loviride: The AVANTI Trial

The AVANTI Trial was an international study in which 106 treatment-naive subjects were randomized to receive ZDV/3TC or ZDV/3TC plus loviride. The median baseline plasma HIV-1 RNA was 63,000 copies/mm^3. After 52 weeks, the HIV-1 RNA decreased by 1.9 log$_{10}$ copies/mm^3 for the double-nucleoside group, versus 2.0 log$_{10}$ copies/mm^3 for those receiving the triple-therapy regimen. Disconcertingly, only 11% of the ZDV/3TC and 20% of the ZDV/3TC/loviride patients had undetectable (<500 copies/mm^3) plasma HIV-1 RNA at 52 weeks. These results were not as encouraging as those from the INCAS Trial, a similar study that used another non-nucleoside, nevirapine, as a component of the treatment regimen.[34]

Use of Non-Nucleoside Reverse Transcriptase Inhibitors With the Protease Inhibitors

Both non-nucleosides and protease inhibitors are metabolized by the liver, and both have effects on the cytochrome P-450 system. These agents therefore will affect the metabolism of other drugs, including one another. Nevirapine and efavirenz (DMP-266) are inducers of this system and, therefore, predictably increase the rate of metabolism for the protease inhibitors, resulting in a decrease in plasma parameters. Delavirdine, on the other hand, inhibits P-450 and would be expected to decrease the rate of metabolism for the protease inhibitors and, therefore, increase plasma parameters. Important issues for clinicians and patients alike are whether these changes are significant, whether they will have any clinical effect, and whether dosages of the drugs should be modified when used concomitantly.

Preliminary data from six pharmacokinetic studies involving nevirapine and delavirdine interactions with the protease inhibitors indinavir (Crixivan®), ritonavir (Norvir®), and saquinavir (Invirase®), were recently presented.

All the nevirapine studies were performed with HIV-1 infected volunteers. No significant interactions between nevirapine and ritonavir were observed. However, there was a respective 28% and 27% decrease in the area under the curve (AUC) of indinavir and saquinavir when nevirapine was coadministered. Although these changes were statistically significant, the question remains whether this is clinically relevant. Preliminary data suggest it is not, at least for indinavir, because the virologic response was significant in magnitude and duration for the combination nevirapine/indinavir administered for up to 32 weeks. The current recommendation is to *consider* increasing the dose of indinavir to 1,000 mg 3 times daily if nevirapine is coadministered. Because the bioavailability of saquinavir in its current formulation is so limited, further reductions in plasma levels, however small, should be avoided. If saquinavir is used with nevirapine, the dose of saquinavir should be increased, perhaps doubled or tripled. Little effect was noted with ritonavir. Interestingly, the protease inhibitors had no effect on nevirapine pharmacokinetics.[36,37]

Delavirdine, which was studied in HIV-1-negative volunteers, had little significant effect on ritonavir pharmacokinetics, although none of the volunteers could tolerate the usual recommended dose of ritonavir. Saquinavir levels, on the other hand, increased by 4- to 6-fold, and indinavir levels by 2-fold. The combination delavirdine/indinavir, 600 mg, was equivalent to 800 mg indinavir as monotherapy. All of the delavirdine/protease inhibitor studies were single dose. As observed with nevirapine, protease inhibitors had no significant effect on delavirdine pharmacokinetic properties.[38]

Only one reported clinical study included a protease inhibitor in a regimen containing a non-nucleoside reverse transcriptase inhibitor. This trial has been informally referred to as the VAN Study, named after Vancouver, the city where

Table 5: Protease Inhibitors: Dosage and Side Effects

Generic Name	Trade Name	Usual Adult Dosage	Side Effects/Comments
indinavir	Crixivan® (Merck)	800 mg q 8 h	kidney stones, must take without food, or with a low-fat, low-protein snack
ritonavir	Norvir® (Abbott)	600 mg b.i.d.	gastrointestinal upset, circumoral paresthesias, many drug interactions
saquinavir	Invirase® (Roche)	600 mg t.i.d.	must take with a fatty snack
nelfinavir	Viracept® (Agouron)	750 mg t.i.d.	diarrhea, must take with food
141W94/ VX-478		1200 mg b.i.d.	experimental

it was performed. In the small, 21-subject, proof-of-concept trial, patients with advanced disease and less than 50 CD4+ cells/mm^3, and extensive prior nucleoside analog therapy but no non-nucleoside or protease inhibitor treatment, received indinavir 800 mg t.i.d., nevirapine 200 mg daily for 2 weeks followed by b.i.d. dosing, plus 3TC 150 mg b.i.d. Patients had a mean baseline CD4+ cell count of 20/mm^3 and mean plasma HIV-1 RNA of 5.12 $\log_{10}$ copies/mm^3.

After 24 weeks, the CD4+ cell counts rose a mean of 75 cells/mm^3, and the plasma HIV-1 RNA decreased by 3.02 $\log_{10}$ copies/mm^3. Fifty-six percent of subjects had plasma HIV-1 RNA levels that decreased below the level of detection (<200/mm^3). The treatment was well tolerated.[39]

This small study was the first trial to use a protease inhibitor with nevirapine, an agent well known to induce cytochrome P-450 isoenzymes and therefore decrease protease levels. Although this was a small, open-label study, it was of interest because there was a robust antiviral response. It did not determine whether the dose or frequency of administration of the protease inhibitor, in this case indinavir, should be altered.

Protease Inhibitor Therapy

HIV-1 protease performs a critical function in the life cycle of HIV-1 by cleaving the polyprotein precursors that ultimately become the core proteins and enzymes of mature virions. Cleavage takes place during the final stages of assembly, while the virion is budding through the host cell membrane. Even if cleavage does not occur, a virion can emerge from the membrane, but this immature particle is incapable of infecting new cells. Unlike reverse transcriptase inhibitors, inhibition of HIV-1 protease directly affects the infected cell pool by halting effective production of new virions.

Once researchers described the structure of the HIV-1 protease enzyme, candidate inhibitors were designed that could bind specifically to the active cleavage site. A dozen pharmaceutical firms have developed hundreds of candidate compounds, of which four have been approved for use in HIV-1 infection: saquinavir, ritonavir, nelfinavir, and indinavir. A fifth, 141W94/VX-478, has entered phase III clinical trials.

The approved protease inhibitors have unquestionably demonstrated potent antiviral, immunologic, and clinical benefits in patients with a variety of HIV-1 disease states. Their effects have been even more pronounced and sustained when used in combination with one or more of the reverse transcriptase inhibitors. The major limitations associated with the use of protease inhibitors are the development of resistance, drug-specific intolerance, and poor penetration into the central nervous system (Table 5).

Unlike resistance to reverse transcriptase, where one critical amino acid substitution can result in phenotypic resistance, resistance to protease inhibitors requires three or more amino acid substitutions and is most likely to occur if the

Table 6: Protease Amino Acid Substitutions in Isolates That Are Resistant

	L10	K20	L24	D30	M36	M46	I47	G48
indinavir	X	X	X		X	X		
ritonavir	X	X				X		
saquinavir	X							
nelfinavir				(X)				X
141W94/VX-478						X	X	

(X) = significant

drugs are used as monotherapy or if viral suppression is incomplete. Resistance patterns overlap considerably between indinavir and ritonavir, but vary somewhat with saquinavir, nelfinavir, and 141W94/VX-478 (Table 6).[40]

Indinavir

Recent clinical endpoint data have been reported that include a survival advantage associated with a regimen containing indinavir (Crixivan®). Indinavir has received accelerated approvals in the USA and other countries based on impressive surrogate marker data.

Indinavir is a potent protease inhibitor with good oral bioavailability when taken on an empty stomach or with a low-fat, low-protein snack. It is dosed at 800 mg every 8 hours in adults. Higher doses show no greater effect and are not as well tolerated. The most important adverse effect associated with indinavir is the development of nephrolithiasis caused by crystallized drug. This occurs in approximately 4% of patients and may be alleviated by aggressive oral hydration. Many patients have been able to continue therapy despite the occasional stone formation. Other side effects include nausea and indirect hyperbilirubinemia, which is typically inconsequential. When administered with two nucleoside analogs, efficacy and duration of effect are enhanced.

I50	I54	L63	A71	V82	I84	N88	L90
	X	X	X	(X)	(X)		X
	X	X	X	(X)	(X)		X
	X	X	X	X	X		(X)
							X
(X)						X	

Two pivotal studies contributed to the licensing approval of indinavir. The Merck 020 Study was an open-label trial comparing indinavir monotherapy with ddI + ZDV and the triple combination indinavir/ddI/ZDV (Table 7). A total of 78 treatment-naive patients with a median $CD4^+$ count at entry of 150 cells/mm^3 and viral RNA of 117,000 copies/mm^3 were enrolled. After 24 weeks, the triple-therapy arm had the most impressive viral load decrease of 3.1 $\log_{10}$ and a $CD4^+$ increase of approximately 100 cells/mm^3. Overall, the triple-therapy patients were more likely to have undetectable amounts of plasma HIV-1 RNA at 24 weeks, 60% compared with 15% for the other groups.[41] Some researchers have suggested that the superior response to the triple therapy was attributable to the limited amount of resistance to both reverse transcriptase and protease compared with that seen in the monotherapy indinavir and combination reverse transcriptase inhibitor groups (Table 7).[42]

The Merck 035 study was a randomized, double-blind trial with 97 adult patients of indinavir monotherapy compared with indinavir/ZDV/3TC and the nucleoside combination of ZDV/3TC. At baseline median, RNA was 41,130 copies/mm^3, and $CD4^+$ was 142 cells/mm^3. All patients had received prior treatment with ZDV, but not with 3TC or a protease inhibitor. After 44 weeks, the median HIV-1 RNA $\log_{10}$ drop was -2.2 log in the triple-therapy arm versus -0.9

Table 7: Development of Resistance by Treatment Arm: Merck 020

	Indinavir Monotherapy	ZDV/ddl Combination Therapy	ZDV/ddl/Indinavir Combination Therapy
AZT- or ddI-associated mutations	1/19	10/16	0/20 $P < 0.001$
indinavir-associated mutations	13/24	1/17	0/20 $P = 0.003$

and -0.2 in the indinavir monotherapy and combination nucleoside arms. Median changes in CD4$^+$ count at 44 weeks were +218, +158, and +14 cells/mm^3 for the three respective groups. The triple-therapy group was most likely to have undetectable amounts of plasma HIV-1 RNA at 44 weeks, 83% versus 22% for the indinavir monotherapy group and 0% in the ZDV/3TC arm (Table 8).[43]

The ACTG 320 trial was a randomized, double-blind, 1,156-subject study comparing ZDV plus 3TC alone versus ZDV, 3TC plus indinavir. Stavudine (d4T) could be substituted for ZDV as needed. Patients were required to have less than 200 CD4$^+$ cells/mm^3 (mean, 86), and have undergone fewer than 7 days of prior 3TC therapy and no prior protease inhibitor treatment. The mean age of the study subjects was 39 years; the population was diverse, and minority groups were well represented. The primary endpoint of this trial was time of progression to an AIDS-defining event or death.[44]

The study was prematurely terminated after a median follow-up of only 38 weeks because significant clinical differences occurred between the indinavir-containing triple-drug regimen arm and the double-nucleoside arm. The rates of progression for the indinavir/ZDV/3TC and ZDV/3TC groups were 6% and 11% [RR=0.50 (95% CI 0.33,0.76;

Table 8: Patients with HIV-1 RNA Below PCR Assay Detection (< 500 copies/mm³): Merck 035 Study

Regimen	Number of Patients (24 weeks)	Number of Patients (32 weeks)	Number of Patients (44 weeks)
IDV+ ZDV+3TC	22/24 (92%)	19/23 (83%)	5/6 (83%)
IDV	9/24 (38%)	8/22 (36%)	2/9 (22%)
ZDV+3TC	0/22 (0%)	0/23 (0%)	0/8 (0%)

$P=0.0010$)]. For the subjects entering the study with less than 50 CD4+ cells/mm³ , the rates of progression were 11% and 20% [RR=0.49 (95% CI 0.30,0.82; $P=0.0051$)]. For those with 51 to 200 CD4+ cells/mm³ , the rates were 3% and 5% [RR=0.51 (95% CI 0.24,1.10; $P=0.080$)]. Eight subjects in the indinavir/ZDV/3TC arm and 18 in the ZDV/3TC arm died (RR=0.43 (95% CI 0.19,0.99; $P=0.042$)].[44]

Overall, the study drugs were well tolerated, with only 10 subjects prematurely discontinuing therapy because of protocol-defined toxicities. The overall study drug discontinuation rate was 20%, which was primarily attributable to subjects' taking open-label protease inhibitors.[44]

The results of this trial clearly demonstrate that adding a protease inhibitor to a nucleoside combination regimen in patients with less than 200/mm³ CD4+ cell counts substantially reduces mortality and clinical disease progression. Because of the results of this large clinical endpoint study, the standard for therapy in this patient group would have to include a protease inhibitor in combination with at least two nucleosides.

Ritonavir

Ritonavir is a potent, orally bioavailable protease inhibitor that has been approved because of promising surrogate marker endpoint data as well as clinical benefits, including a survival advantage observed in one study. Ritonavir is dosed 600 mg twice daily and may be taken with or without food.

The 100-mg gelcaps must be refrigerated. The main problems associated with ritonavir are gastrointestinal intolerance, circumoral paresthesias, and significant drug interactions from its nearly complete inhibition of the CYP3A4 hepatic isoenzyme. Adverse effects can be minimized when initiating therapy if the dosage is gradually increased over the first 2 weeks.

Full approval for ritonavir was granted because of the survival advantage observed in Abbott Study 247. In this trial, 1,090 patients with extensive prior antiretroviral treatment and CD4+ cell counts below 100/mm^3 were randomized to receive ritonavir or placebo in addition to their therapy of zero, one, or two nucleoside analog reverse transcriptase inhibitors. After a median of 6.1 months, 4.8% of the patients receiving ritonavir had died versus 8.4% of those on placebo (P=0.02). There was a similar benefit observed in delay of disease progression. Drug discontinuation associated with adverse events occurred in 17% of the ritonavir patients versus 6% for those taking placebo. Patients taking concomitant anti-HIV-1 treatment did better than those who did not.[45]

Another trial using ritonavir was a 12-patient, open-label study of combination ritonavir/ZDV/3TC in individuals with recently acquired HIV-1 infection. An interim analysis of this ongoing study demonstrated that, in nearly all cases, HIV-1 was undetectable when measured by PBMC coculture and by plasma RNA. CD4+ counts rose substantially and the CD4+/CD8 count returned to normal. Therapy is planned to continue for 1 year, when a lymph node biopsy will be performed and assessed for the presence of active viral replication. A decision will then be made whether to stop therapy.[46]

Saquinavir

Saquinavir was the first protease inhibitor to be approved for use in HIV-1 infection. Although a well-tolerated drug, oral bioavailability is poor, with only 4% being absorbed when taken with a fatty snack. Without food, virtually none is absorbed. The current recommended dosage is 600 mg 3 times daily. Newer suspension formulations at higher doses are being studied, as are combinations with other protease inhibitors such as ritonavir, which inhibit saquinavir metabolism and result in significantly higher plasma levels of saquinavir.

Saquinavir was approved because of moderately impressive surrogate marker data. Since then, clinical endpoint data have suggested a survival advantage for patients receiving saquinavir plus ddC.[47,48]

The first major study of saquinavir was the ACTG 229 trial that compared saquinavir + ZDV versus saquinavir + ZDV + ddC versus ZDV + ddC. In this double-blind trial of 302 treatment-experienced patients with counts of 50 to 300 CD4$^+$ cells/mm^3, the normalized area under the curve for the CD4$^+$ cell count was greater with the three-drug combination, as was the reduction in plasma HIV-1 RNA. These benefits were not sustained over time, however, and the saquinavir + ZDV group appeared to respond the poorest.[47]

More impressive data have been reported from the NV14256 Study. In this trial, 978 patients with a CD4$^+$ count between 50 and 300 cells/mm^3 and a minimum of 16 weeks of prior ZDV therapy were randomized in a double-blind fashion to receive ddC or saquinavir monotherapy versus the combination of both. The combination did the best, as expected. Both for the time to first AIDS-defining event or death and for survival alone, statistically significant benefits favored the combination over ddC. No significant differences were found in the comparison of saquinavir to ddC.[48] This study has been criticized because of the expected weakness of the monotherapy arms.

Saquinavir Plus Ritonavir

The major problem associated with saquinavir is the poor plasma levels that are achieved with a standard oral dosage of 600 mg 3 times daily. This can be significantly altered if saquinavir is given in combination with ritonavir, a potent inhibitor of saquinavir metabolism. Plasma levels of saquinavir in the presence of ritonavir are approximately 60-fold higher than when given alone. Preliminary results of a pilot study where both drugs were given together indicate that there is a significant rise in $CD4^+$ count and a drop in HIV-1 RNA. The study has now covered only 24 weeks, but the combination appeared fairly well tolerated except for the expected adverse events associated with ritonavir and grade IV hepatic enzyme elevations noted in patients with chronic hepatitis C or B.[49] Until this study is completed and the full safety profile known, this combination should be used cautiously.

Nelfinavir

Nelfinavir (Viracept®) is the most recently approved protease inhibitor, available for children and adults. Nelfinavir appears to be well tolerated, the only significant reported adverse effect being mild diarrhea, which occurs in up to 30% of patients. The recommended dosage is 750 mg taken 3 times daily with food. Preliminary results have been reported from four trials.

In Agouron Study 506, nelfinavir 500 mg and 750 mg given 3 times daily with d4T, 40 mg twice daily, was administered to 307 patients with more than 50 $CD4^+$ cells/mm³ (mean, 279) and more than 15,000 copies/mm³ (mean, 141,400) of plasma HIV-1 RNA. No patients had ever received a protease inhibitor or d4T; 20% were antiretroviral naive at study entry. At 24 weeks, the plasma HIV-1 RNA decrease from baseline was approximately 0.7 $\log_{10}$ copies/mm³ for d4T, and 1.0 and 1.1 $\log_{10}$ copies/mm³ for the two nelfinavir-containing arms. The $CD4^+$ cell counts increased by 106 and 103/mm³ in the nelfinavir arms, versus 51/mm³ in the d4T monotherapy group. Nineteen percent and 20% of the nelfinavir-group patients, and only 2% of those receiving d4T, experienced a decrease in plasma HIV-1 RNA below detection levels.[49]

Protocols 511 and 509: More impressive results have been reported in a treatment-naive, 297-patient trial of nelfinavir, 500 mg or 750 mg 3 times daily plus ZDV/3TC, versus ZDV/3TC alone. There was no $CD4^+$ cell count restriction (mean, 288/mm³) and plasma HIV-1 RNA had to be greater than 15,000 copies/mm^3 (mean, 153,000). After 24 weeks, plasma HIV-1 RNA decreased by 1.9 log$_{10}$, 2.0 log$_{10}$, and 1.4 log$_{10}$ copies/mm^3, while CD4$^+$ cell counts increased by 161/mm^3, 155/mm^3, and 105/mm^3. More of the patients in the higher-dose nelfinavir arm experienced plasma HIV-1 RNA decrease to below the level of detection (500 copies/mm^3), 81% versus 65%. Only 18% of subjects assigned to receive ZDV/3TC experienced a decrease in plasma HIV-1 RNA to undetectable levels.[50] Because of this finding, the 750-mg nelfinavir dosage was approved for marketing purposes in the United States.

In another trial, nelfinavir plus ZDV and 3TC was given in combination to 12 antiretroviral-naive patients who were chronically infected with HIV-1. After 3 months of open-label treatment, 11 patients had undetectable plasma HIV-1 RNA and were negative in PBMC cocultures. The median increase in CD4$^+$ at 12 weeks was 98 cells/mm^3. One patient dropped out because of a grade 4 elevation of CPK and moderate diarrhea.[51]

Nelfinavir is a promising potent protease inhibitor. However, the resistance profile compared with the profile of the other approved agents in its class, may overlap significantly.

141W94/VX-478

141W94/VX-478 is another protease inhibitor. Data exist on 55 patients who have taken the drug for 28 days as monotherapy in a dose-escalation study or in conjunction with abacavir (1592U89), a new nucleoside analog. None of these patients had ever previously received a protease inhibitor. The results of this trial demonstrate a dose response favoring the highest dose tested, 1,200 mg twice daily. At this dosage, a -1.95 log$_{10}$ median maximal change from baseline in plasma HIV-1 RNA and a 110 CD4$^+$ cell increase were observed. Adverse experiences occurring in more than 10% of patients included mild rash, diarrhea, and headache. Two patients discontinued therapy because of rash and another one because of worsening colitis. One case of Stevens-Johnson syndrome has been reported.[52,53]

The future development of this compound will include combination studies with at least two nucleoside analog reverse transcriptase inhibitors.

Conclusions

The obvious goal of treating HIV-1 infection is to eradicate the infection, and if that is not possible, to reduce the viral burden by as much as possible, allowing the immune system to recover. These, we hope, will delay disease progression and improve survival. We know we can eradicate infection if therapy is started very early, such as with treatment after accidental occupational exposure and with neonates who are treated in utero, during labor, and for several weeks after birth. Infection rates in these two cases drops by 66% to 80% compared with those that are untreated.[54,55] It remains to be seen whether treating any other group of patients, including those who have only recently become infected, will ever be cured, although studies are in progress.

The next best treatment we can offer patients is one that they can tolerate and that maximally reduces the circulating viral burden. This means a regimen that decreases plasma HIV-1 RNA to undetectable amounts. The only regimens that have been associated with this type of response so far have involved three drugs from two different categories of agents: nucleoside reverse transcriptase inhibitors plus a protease inhibitor or non-nucleoside reverse transcriptase inhibitor. If this is impossible, a drop in plasma HIV-1 RNA of at least $0.5 \log_{10}$ is essential.

In patients who fail to respond to initial therapy, the ideal option is to replace the entire treatment regimen with agents that might be sensitive. For example, ZDV may become resensitized when 3TC is added. Clinicians must keep in mind that protease inhibitors, as well as the non-nucleoside reverse transcriptase inhibitors, may have significantly overlapping resistance patterns. Updated recommendations regarding therapy for adult patients with HIV-1 infection have recently been published. Clinicians should review these rec-

Table 10: Treatment Recommendations: 1997 Triple-Therapy Options (choose one from each column)

Nucleoside #1	Nucleoside #2	Protease inhibitor or NNRTI
zidovudine	didanosine	indinavir
stavudine	zalcitabine*	nelfinavir
	lamivudine	ritonavir
		nevirapine

* Zalcitabine plus stavudine has not been studied, and may be toxic.

ommendations before initiating antiretroviral therapy, or when considering changing a patient's regimen.

Initiating therapy should be considered early in the infectious course and treatment should be aggressive. Whether there is a role for combination nucleoside reverse transcriptase inhibitor regimens by themselves is in question. At a minimum, monotherapy with any agent should be avoided, as should dose interruptions and dosage reductions in the protease and non-nucleoside classes of agents.[1,56] Table 10 provides a guideline for choosing an antiretroviral regimen. This is expected to change as newer and more powerful therapies become available.

References

1.   Carpenter CC, Fischl MA, Hammer SM, et al: Antiretroviral therapy for HIV infection in 1997. International AIDS Society—USA. *JAMA* 1997;277:1962-1969.

2.   Concorde Coordinating Committee Panel: MRC/ANRS randomised double-blind controlled trial of immediate and deferred zidovudine in symptom-free HIV infection. *Lancet* 1994;343:871-881.

3.   Volberding PA, Lagakos SW, Grimes JM, et al: A comparison of immediate with deferred zidovudine therapy for asymptomatic HIV-infected adults with CD4 cell counts of 500 or more per cubic millimeter. AIDS Clinical Trials Group. *N Engl J Med* 1995;333:401-407.

4.   Hammer SM, Katzenstein DA, Hughes MD, et al: A trial comparing nucleoside monotherapy with combination therapy in HIV-infected adults with CD4 cell counts from 200 to 500 per cubic millimeter. *N Engl J Med* 1996;335:1081-1090.

5.   Delta Coordinating Committee: A randomised double-blind controlled trial comparing combinations of zidovudine plus didanosine or zalcitabine with zidovudine alone in HIV-infected individuals. *Lancet* 1996;348:283-291.

6.   Saravolatz LD, Winslow DL, Collins G, et al: Zidovudine alone or in combination with didanosine or zalcitabine in HIV-infected patients with the acquired immunodeficiency syndrome or fewer than 200 CD4 cells per cubic millimeter. Investigators for the Terry Beirn Community Programs for Clinical Research on AIDS. *N Engl J Med* 1996;335:1099-1106.

7.   Eron JJ, Benoit SL, Jemsek J, et al: Treatment with lamivudine, zidovudine, or both in HIV-positive patients with 200 to 500 CD4+ cells per cubic millimeter. North American HIV Working Party. *N Engl J Med* 1995;333:1662-1669.

8.   Katlama C, Ingrand D, Loveday C, et al: Safety and efficacy of lamivudine-zidovudine combination therapy in antiretroviral-naive patients. A randomized controlled comparison with zidovudine monotherapy. *JAMA* 1996;276:118-125.

9.   Staszewski S, Loveday C, Picazo JJ, et al: Safety and efficacy of lamivudine-zidovudine combination therapy in zidovudine-experienced patients. A randomized controlled comparison with zidovudine monotherapy. Lamivudine European HIV Working Group. *JAMA* 1996;276:111-117.

10. Bartlett JA, Benoit SL, Johnson VA, et al: Lamivudine plus zidovudine compared with zalcitabine plus zidovudine in patients with HIV infection. A randomized, double-blind, placebo-controlled trial. North American HIV Working Party. *Ann Intern Med* 1996;125:161-172.

11. Larder BA, Kemp SD, Harrigan PR: Potential mechanism for sustained antiretroviral efficacy of AZT-3TC combination therapy. *Science* 1995;269:696-699.

12. CAESAR Coordinating Committee. Randomised trial of addition of lamivudine or lamivudine plus loviride to zidovudine-containing regimens for patients with HIV-1 infection: the CAESAR trial. *Lancet* 1997;349:1413-1421.

13. Rouleau D, Conway B, Raboud J, et al: A pilot, open-label study of the antiviral effect of stavudine (d4T) and lamivudine (3TC) in ad-

vanced HIV disease. 11th International Conference on AIDS, Vancouver, 1996. Abstract We.B.3137.

14. Katlama C, Valantin MA, Calvez V, et al: ALTIS: a pilot study of d4T/3TC in antiretroviral naive and experienced patients. In: Abstracts of the 4th Conferece on Retroviruses and Opportunistic Infections. Washington, DC: January 22-26, 1997, abstract LB4.

15. Pollard R, Peterson D, Hardy D, et al: Stavudine (d4T) and didanosine (ddI) combination therapy in HIV-infected subjects: antiviral effect and safety in an on-going pilot, randomized double-blinded trial. 11th International Conference on AIDS, Vancouver, 1996. Abstract Th.B.293.

16. Raffi F, Auger S, Billaud E, et al: Antiviral effect and safety of didanosine-stavudine combination therapy in HIV-infected subjects: interim results of a pilot trial. In: Abstracts of the 4th Conference on Retroviruses and Opportunistic Infections. Washington, DC: January 22-26, 1997, abstract 554.

17. Durant J, Rahelinirina V, Delmas B, et al: A pilot study of the combination of stavudine (d4T) and didanosine (ddI) in patients with <350 CD4/mm^3 and who are not eligible for a treatment with ZDV. In: Abstracts of the 4th Conference on Retroviruses and Opportunistic Infections. Washington, DC: January 22-26, 1997, abstract 553.

18. Gu Z, Quan Y, Li Z, et al: Effects of non-nucleoside inhibitors of human immunodeficiency virus type 1 in cell-free recombinant reverse transcriptase assays. *J Biol Chem* 1995;270:31,046-31,051.

19. Smerdon SJ, Jager J, Wang J, et al: Structure of the binding site for non-nucleoside inhibitors of the reverse transcriptase of human immunodeficiency virus type 1. *Proc Natl Acad Sci U S A* 1994; 26:3911-3915.

20. Ding J, Das K, Moereels H, et al: Structure of HIV-1 TR/TIBO R 86183 complex reveals similarity in the binding of diverse nonnucleoside inhibitors. *Nat Struct Biol* 1995;2:407-415.

21. Murphy RL, Montaner J: Nevirapine: a review of its development, pharmacological profile and potential for clinical use. *Exp Opin Invest Drugs* 1996;5:1183-1199.

22. Merrill DP, Moonis M, Chou TC, et al: Lamivudine or stavudine in two- and three-drug combinations against human immunodeficiency virus type 1 replication in vitro. *J Infect Dis* 1996;173:355-364.

23. St. Clair MH, Pennington KN, Rooney J, et al: In vitro comparison of selected triple-drug combinations for suppression of HIV-1

replication: the Inter-Company Collaboration Protocol. *J Acquir Immune Defic Syndr Hum Retrovirol* 1995;10(suppl 2):S83-S91.

24. Koup RA, Brewster F, Grob P, et al: Nevirapine synergistically inhibits HIV-1 replication in combination with zidovudine, interferon or CD4 immunoadhesin. *AIDS* 1993;7:1181-1184.

25. Havlir D, McLaughlin MM, Richman DD: A pilot study to evaluate the development of resistance to nevirapine in asymptomatic human immunodeficiency virus-infected patients with CD4 cell counts of >500/mm^3: AIDS Clinical Trials Group Protocol 208. *J Infect Dis* 1995;172:1379-1383.

26. Myers MW, Montaner JG: The INCAS Study Group: A randomized, double-blind comparative trial of the effects of zidovudine, didanosine, and nevirapine combinations in antiviral-naive, AIDS-free, HIV-infected patients with CD4 counts 200 to 600/mm^3. In: Abstracts of the 11th International Conference on AIDS, Vancouver, 1996. Abstract Mo.B.294.

27. D'Aquila RT, Hughes MD, Johnson VA, et al: Nevirapine, zidovudine, and didanosine compared with zidovudine and didanosine in patients with HIV-1 infection. A randomized, double-blind, placebo-controlled trial. National Institute of Allergy and Infectious Diseases AIDS Clinical Trials Group Protocol 241 Investigators. *Ann Intern Med* 1996;124:1019-1030.

28. Henry K, Thierny C, Kahn J, et al: A randomized, double-blind placebo-controlled study comparing combination nucleoside and triple therapy for the treatment of advanced HIV disease (CD4 <50/mm^3). In: Abstracts of the 4th Conference on Retroviruses and Opportunistic Infections. Washington, DC: January 22-26, 1997, abstract LB6.

29. In a conversation with M. Myers, Boehringer Ingelheim Pharmaceuticals, Ridgefield, CT.

30. Freimuth WW, Chuang-Stein CJ, Greenwald CA, et al: Delavirdine (DLV) combined with zidovudine (ZDV) or didanosine (ddI) produces sustained reduction in viral burden and increases in CD4 counts in early and advanced HIV-1 infection. In: Abstracts of the 11th International Conference on AIDS, Vancouver, 1996. Abstract Mo.B. 295.

31. Freimuth WW, Chuang-Stein CJ, Greenwald C, et al: Delavirdine (DLV) + didanosine (ddI) combination therapy has sustained surrogate marker response in advanced HIV-1 populations. In: Abstracts of the 3rd Conference on Retroviruses and Opportunistic Infections. Washington, DC: January 28-February 1, 1996, abstract LB8b.

32. Medical and Drug Information Unit, Pharmacia & Upjohn: Comprehensive Review of Rescriptor, April 24, 1997.

33. Staszewski S, Miller V, Kober A, et al: Evaluation of the efficacy and tolerance of RO 18893, RO 89439 (loviride) and placebo in asymptomatic HIV-1 infected patients. *Antiviral Ther* 1996;1:42-50.

34. Rozenbaum W: AVANTI 1: a randomized, double-blind, comparative trial to evaluate the efficacy, safety and tolerance of combination antiretroviral regimens for the treatment of HIV infection. In: Abstracts of the 4th Conference on Retroviruses and Opportunistic Infections. Washington, DC: January 22-26, 1997, abstract 368.

36. Murphy RL, Gagnier P, Lamson M, et al: Effect of nevirapine on pharmacokinetics of indinavir and ritonavir in HIV-1 patients. In: Abstracts of the 4th Conference on Retroviruses and Opportunistic Infections. Washington, DC: January 22-26, 1997, abstract 372.

37. Sahai J, Cameron W, Salgo M, et al: Drug interaction study between saquinavir and nevirapine. In: Abstracts of the 4th Conference on Retroviruses and Opportunisitic Infections. Washington, DC: January 22-26, 1997, abstract 614.

38. Cox SR, Ferry JJ, Batts DH, et al: Delavirdine and marketed protease inhibitors: pharmacokinetic interaction studies in health volunteers. In: Abstracts of the 4th Conference on Retroviruses and Opportunistic Infections. Washington, DC: January 22-26, 1997, abstract 372.

39. Harris M, Durakovic C, Conway B, et al: A pilot study of indinavir, nevirapine, and 3TC in patients with advanced HIV disease. In: Abstracts of the 4th Conference on Retroviruses and Opportunistic Infections. Washington, DC: January 22-26, 1997, abstract 234.

40. Condra JH, Schleif WA, Blahy OM, et al: In vivo emergence of IIIV-1 variants resistant to multiple protease inhibitors. *Nature* 1995;374:569-571.

41. Massari R, Conant M, Mellors J, et al: A phase II open-label randomized study of the triple combination of indinavir, zidovudine (ZDV) and didanosine (DDI) versus indinavir alone and zidovudine/didanosine in antiretroviral naive patients. In: Abstracts of the 3rd Conference on Retroviruses and Opportunistic Infections. Washington, DC: 1996, abstract 200.

42. Condra JH, Holder DJ, Schleif WA, et al: Bi-directional inhibition of HIV-1 drug resistance selection by combination therapy with indinavir and reverse transcriptase inhibitors. In: Abstracts of the 11th International Conference on AIDS, Vancouver, 1996. Abstract Th.B.932.

43. Gulick R, Mellors J, Havlir D, et al: Potent and sustained antiretroviral activity of indinavir (IND), zidovudine (ZDV) and lamivudine (3TC). In: Abstracts of the 11th International Conference on AIDS, Vancouver, 1996. Abstract Th.B.931.

44. Hammer SM, Squires KE, Hughes MD, et al: A controlled trial of two nucleoside analogues plus indinavir in persons with human immunodeficiency virus infection and CD4 cell counts of 200 per cubic millimeter or less. *N Engl J Med* 1997;337:725-733.

45. Cameron DW, Heath-Chiozzi M, Kravick SI, et al: Prolongation of life and prevention of AIDS complications in advanced HIV immunodeficiency with ritonavir: update. In: Abstracts of the 11th International Conference on AIDS, Vancouver, 1996. Abstract Mo.B.411.

46. Markowitz M, Cao Y, Hurley A, et al: Triple therapy with AZT, 3TC, and ritonavir in 12 subjects newly infected with HIV-1. In: Abstracts of the 11th International Conference on AIDS. Vancouver, 1996. Abstract Th.B.933.

47. Collier AC, Coombs RW, Schoenfeld DA, et al: Treatment of human immunodeficiency virus infection with saquinavir, zidovudine, and zalcitabine. AIDS Clinical Trials Group. *N Engl J Med* 1996;334:1011-1017.

48. Lalezari J, Haubrich R, Burger HU, et al: Improved survival and decreased progression of HIV in patients treated with saquinavir (Invirase™, SQV) plus HIVID (zalcitabine, ddC). In: Abstracts of the 11th International Conference on AIDS. Vancouver, 1996. Abstract LB.B.6033.

49. Cohen C, Sun E, Cameron W, et al: Ritonavir-saquinavir combination treatment in HIV-infected patients. In: Abstracts of the 36th Interscience Conference on Antimicrobial Agents and Chemotherapy, New Orleans, 1996. Abstract LB07B.

50. Powderly W, Sension M, Conant M, et al: The efficacy of Viracept (nelfinavir mesylate, NLF) in pivotal phase II/III double-blind randomized controlled trials as monotherapy and in combination with d4T or AZT/3TC. In: Abstracts of the 4th Conference on Retroviruses and Opportunistic Infections. Washington, DC: January 22-26, 1997, abstract 370.

51. Markowitz M, Cao Y, Hurley A, et al: Triple therapy with AZT and 3TC in combination with nelfinavir mesylate in 12 antiretroviral-naive subjects chronically infected with HIV-1. In: Abstracts of the 11th International Conference on AIDS, Vancouver, 1996. Abstract LB.B.6031.

52. Schooley RT: Preliminary data on the safety and antiviral efficacy of the novel protease inhibitor 141W94 in HIV-infected patients with 150-400 CD4 cells/mm³. In: Abstracts of the 36th Interscience Conference on Antimicrobial Agents and Chemotherapy. New Orleans: September 15-18, 1996. abstract LB07a.

53. Schooley RT: Preliminary data from a phase I/II study on the safety and antiviral efficacy of the combination of 141W94 plus 1592U89 in HIV-infected patients with 150-400 CD4+ cells/mm³. In: Abstracts of the 4th Conference on Retroviruses and Opportunistic Infections. Washington, DC: January 22-26, 1997, abstract LB3.

54. Connor EM, Sperling RS, Gelber R, et al: Reduction of maternal-infant transmission of human immunodeficiency virus type 1 with zidovudine treatment. Pediatric AIDS Clinical Trials Group Protocol 076 Study Group. *N Engl J Med* 1994;331:1173-1180.

55. US Public Health Service: Update: provisional Public Health Service recommendations for chemoprophylaxis after occupational exposure to HIV. *MMWR Morb Mortal Wkly Rep* 1996;45:468-480.

56. Saag MS, Holodniy M, Kuritzkes DR, et al: HIV viral load markers in clinical practice. *Nat Med* 1996;2:625-629.

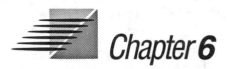 *Chapter 6*

Prevention of Opportunistic Infections

Clinical experience in the 1970s demonstrated that trimethoprim/sulfamethoxazole (TMP/SMX) could be used to prevent *Pneumocystis carinii* pneumonia (PCP) in children receiving aggressive chemotherapy for acute lymphocytic leukemia and rhabdomyosarcoma. By the mid-1980s, this discovery led to efforts to prevent PCP in HIV-1 infected patients, the most common initial AIDS-defining event. Chemoprophylaxis with TMP/SMX or with periodic administration of aerosolized pentamidine (NebuPent®) was soon documented to reduce the prevalence of PCP in patients with advanced HIV-1 infection.[1,2] In addition, analysis of the occurrence of PCP in the Multicenter AIDS Cohort Study (MACS) demonstrated that HIV-1 infected individuals with less than 200/mm³ of CD4+ lymphocytes were at increased risk of developing PCP.[3] Men with higher CD4+ lymphocyte counts but with sustained fever or thrush were also at increased risk of developing this complication.[4] When research demonstrated that prophylaxis could reduce PCP prevalence and when a subpopulation of HIV-1 infected persons was easily identified who would benefit from treatment, the U.S. Public Health Service released the first of a series of recommendations about the prevention of PCP in adults and children.[5-9]

Table 1: Recommended Prophylaxis Measures to Prevent Opportunistic Infections

Condition	Prophylaxis
Pneumocystis carinii pneumonia • CD4+ count less than 200/mm³ • unexplained fever (>100°F) for ≥2 weeks • history of oropharyngeal candidiasis	First Line • TMP/SMX single or double strength daily Second Line • TMP/SMX double strength 3/week • dapsone 100 mg daily • atovaquone suspension 1,500 mg daily • aerosolized pentamidine 300 mg monthly
Disseminated MAC • CD4+ count less than 50/mm³	First Line • clarithromycin 500 mg b.i.d. • azithromycin 1,200 mg weekly Second Line • rifabutin 300 mg daily • rifabutin 150 mg daily with indinavir therapy
Tuberculosis Positive skin test with purified protein derivative • all HIV-infected patients	• isoniazid 300 mg daily plus pyridoxine 50 mg daily x 12 months
Toxoplasma gondii cerebritis • positive IgG antibody to _Toxoplasma gondii_ • CD4+ count less than 100/mm³	First Line • TMP/SMX DS daily Second Line • pyrimethamine 50 mg plus folinic acid 15 mg weekly plus dapsone 100 mg daily • atovaquone suspension 1,500 mg daily

Subsequently, additional information about reducing the risk of exposure and recommendations for preventing other opportunistic infections have been promulgated by the Centers for Disease Control and Prevention, the National Institutes of Health, and the Infectious Disease Society of America.[8,9] Table 1 outlines the current recommendations for prevention of selected opportunistic infections. This chapter reviews these recommendations and the clinical information on which they are based.

Pneumocystis carinii Pneumonia Prophylaxis

The impact of PCP prophylaxis has been documented in several observational studies.[10,11] In the Multicenter AIDS Cohort Study (MACS), the study participants receiving PCP prophylaxis had an approximate 50% reduction in the incidence of PCP as the initial AIDS-defining event compared with patients with less than $200/mm^3$ CD4+ cell count who had not been given prophylaxis. Among those receiving prophylaxis, CD4+ cell counts were lower in persons who developed PCP, compared with persons not receiving prophylaxis. The authors suggested that PCP prophylaxis resulted in a gain of 6 to 9 months of AIDS-free time. The most common AIDS-defining infections in those receiving prophylaxis included disseminated *Mycobacterium avium* complex (MAC) infection, cytomegalovirus disease, and invasive fungal infections.[10]

In an attempt to find the most effective method of preventing PCP, the AIDS Clinical Trials Group (ACTG) undertook a trial to compare trimethoprim/sulfamethoxazole (TMP/SMX, Bactrim®, Septra®), dapsone, and aerosolized pentamidine.[11] Analysis based on intention-to-treat demonstrated no major difference in the effectiveness of these three forms of prophylaxis. However, an on-treatment analysis demonstrated that systemic prophylaxis was superior to aerosolized pentamidine. Very few patients receiving TMP/SMX developed PCP while on therapy. TMP/SMX was associated with the highest prevalence of adverse events, primarily rash and fever, which required a frequent change to dapsone or aerosolized pentamidine.[12]

In other studies, aerosolized pentamidine, a form of topical therapy, was effective in preventing PCP but was associated with extrapulmonary pneumocystosis, which provided more evidence for the value of systemic therapy.[13] Recently, atovaquone suspension 1,500 mg daily was shown to be as effective as dapsone 100 mg daily in patients intolerant to TMP/SMX. With further experience, all forms of PCP prophylaxis have been shown to provide incomplete protection against development of this complication of HIV-1 infection. Patients who develop "breakthrough" PCP are generally those with far-advanced immunosuppression, typically with $CD4^+$ cell counts less than $50/mm^3$ and who often have had other infectious or neoplastic complications.[14] If tolerated, the most effective form of prophylaxis for PCP is generally felt to be TMP/SMX, administered daily or 3 times per week.

Toxoplasmosis

The daily administration of TMP/SMX also provides prophylaxis for a second infectious complication of HIV-1-induced immunosuppression, *Toxoplasma gondii* cerebritis.[15] One study suggested that a similar level of protection against reactivation of this protozoan infection in *Toxoplasma gondii* antibody-positive patients was provided by a regimen of TMP/SMX administered twice a week.[16] Seropositive individuals who cannot tolerate TMP/SMX are at risk for developing toxoplasmosis when their $CD4^+$ lymphocyte count falls below $100/mm^3$.

Pyrimethamine (Daraprim®) given with folinic acid in combination with dapsone is an effective prophylaxis therapy for toxoplasmosis. In a multinational trial, this combination reduced the incidence of cerebritis from this organism if patients could tolerate the agents and remain on treatment. Pyrimethamine plus folinic acid alone was not effective.[17]

Initially, it was felt that TMP/SMX also provided prophylaxis for bacterial infections caused by *Streptococcus pneumoniae* and *Haemophilus influenzae*. However, within the last year an increasing number of TMP/SMX-resistant *S pneumoniae* have been identified in the HIV-1 infected and general populations,[18] which decreases the use of this agent as a means of preventing bacterial infection. Recently, data from a large trial suggested that atovaquone suspension, 1,500 mg daily, may prevent the development of toxoplasmosis. Patients receiving this regimen had very low rates of toxoplasmosis, comparable to patients who received dapsone plus pyrimethamine and folinic acid.

Mycobacterium avium Complex (MAC) Disease

Two macrolide antibiotics, clarithromycin (Biaxin®)[19] and azithromycin (Zithromax®),[20] effectively reduce the occurrence of MAC infection in similar populations. Furthermore, the combination of 1,200 mg of azithromycin once per week, plus daily rifabutin was more effective but not as well tolerated than either drug given alone. Breakthrough MAC infection that occurred in patients who received the macrolides alone was attributed to resistant organisms complicating the treatment of these infections.

Disseminated MAC infection occurs with increasing frequency in persons with less than $50/mm^3$ CD4$^+$ lymphocytes. Two trials, one conducted in the United States and the other in Canada, demonstrated that rifabutin (Mycobutin®) at 300 mg per day reduced the occurrence of MAC infection by 50% in persons with less than $200/mm^3$ CD4$^+$ cells.[19-21] Interestingly, "breakthrough" infections were not caused by rifabutin-resistant mycobacteria. These initial studies failed to demonstrate a survival benefit associated with prevention of MAC. However, follow-up analysis indicated that rifabutin prophylaxis prolonged life in patients with less than and more than $50/mm^3$ CD4$^+$ lymphocytes.[19] The results of the original trials led to the initial 1993 recommendation by the U.S. Public Health Service to administer rifabutin to all HIV-1 infected individuals with less than $75/mm^3$ CD4$^+$ lymphocytes.[20]

Rifabutin prophylaxis raises additional issues relevant to the management of patients with advanced HIV-1 infection. This rifamycin agent induces the hepatic cytochrome

P-450 3A enzyme system, which potentially leads to several important drug interactions that can complicate therapy of such patients. The combination of the triazole antifungal agent fluconazole (Diflucan®) and rifabutin produces increasing plasma concentrations of rifabutin and subsequent toxicity, primarily uveitis. Because of its metabolism by this hepatic enzyme system, rifabutin must be used at half dose when the protease inhibitor indinavir (Crixivan®) is administered. It is contraindicated with use of ritonavir (Norvir®).[24]

Candidiasis

Esophageal candidiasis and oropharyngeal candidiasis can be prevented by daily administration of fluconazole.[25] However, routine prophylaxis with this agent is not recommended because of the effectiveness of therapy for acute disease, the low mortality associated with mucosal candidiasis, and the potential for azole resistance. Infection with fluconazole-resistant fungi such as *Aspergillus fumigatis*, non-albicans *Candida*, and resistant *Candida albicans* are not prevented or are increased in prevalence with chronic use of fluconazole.[26] Therefore, prophylaxis for candidiasis is generally not recommended.

Cryptococcosis

Itraconazole and fluconazole can decrease the incidence of cryptococcal disease in patients with less than 50 CD4+ cells/mm^3. However, routine use of either agent is not recommended because of high cost and lack of survival benefit associated with prophylaxis.[25]

Histoplasmosis

Itraconazole should be considered for patients with less than 100 CD4+ cells/mm^3 who live in an area that is endemic for *Histoplasma capsulatum*.

Coccidioidomycosis

No recommendation can be made regarding prophylaxis for persons living in coccidioidomycosis-endemic areas or for persons who skin test positive and live in nonendemic areas.

Cytomegalovirus Infections

Prolongation of survival with more effective antiretroviral therapy and widespread administration of PCP prophylaxis has resulted in an increasing prevalence of cytomegalovirus (CMV) disease. Sight-threatening retinitis is the most common manifestation of this viral infection, although CMV esophagitis, colitis, hepatitis, pneumonia, encephalitis, and myelitis also occur in persons with advanced HIV-1 infection. Approximately 40% of patients with CD4+ lymphocyte counts below 50/mm^3 will develop CMV retinitis.[26]

Two large prophylactic trials of oral ganciclovir (Cytovene®) have been conducted; the first clearly demonstrated a reduction in the prevalence of CMV disease but was not associated with prolongation of survival. The second did not demonstrate any benefit. The first trial used periodic, routine retinal photography and was conducted for a longer time, although the patient populations enrolled in the two trials were similar.[27,28] Ganciclovir suppresses the bone marrow, often requiring the use of granulocyte colony-stimulating factor, requires the ingestion of many pills each day, and is expensive. Thus, finding a less toxic, less expensive, more user-friendly regimen in a well-defined population at risk is necessary.

The ACTG 204 trial evaluated the use of valacyclovir (Valtrex®) as a method of preventing this severe viral complication of HIV-1 infection. Valacyclovir was compared to high (800 mg 5 times per day) and routine dosages of acyclovir (Zovirax®), 400 mg twice daily. The participants who received valacyclovir had a significantly reduced occurrence of CMV disease, but a trend toward increased mortality.[29] Both the first oral ganciclovir trial and the ACTG 204 trial conducted substudies that suggested that the subset of individuals with CMV viremia at baseline appeared to benefit from prophylaxis.[30,31] These individuals were apparently receiving preemptive therapy, analogous to treatment of recent PPD skin test converters with isoniazid (INH; Nydrazid®, Rifamate®).

The patients with advanced HIV-1 infection who are at increased risk of developing CMV disease remain to be definitively identified. Patients with disseminated MAC appear to be at great risk of developing CMV disease and, conversely, patients with CMV are vulnerable to disseminated MAC.[32] This may be because of the high prevalence of both diseases in patients with advanced HIV-1 infection. Alternatively, this association could be caused by enhanced immunosuppression produced by HIV-1 replication augmented by the complicating infections or by the direct effects of the mycobacterial or herpetic virus infection on cell-mediated immunity.

Tuberculosis

Finally, all persons diagnosed with HIV-1 infection should be skin tested with intermediate-strength purified protein derivative (PPD) as early as possible. All HIV-1 infected persons with PPD reactions with 5 mm or more of induration should receive INH prophylaxis, 300 mg per day, plus pyridoxine, 50 mg daily, for 12 months. Homeless individuals, injection drug users, and HIV-1 infected persons exposed to *Mycobacterium tuberculosis* who are anergic should also receive INH prophylaxis.[33]

Risk Reduction

For many HIV-1 related opportunistic infections, prophylaxis is not available or has yet to be proven effective. Therefore, prevention of exposure is the most effective means of reducing the risk of infection. Examples include boiling tap water to prevent cryptosporidiosis if there is an indication that the water supply has been contaminated,[34] reducing exposure to kittens to reduce the risk of *Bartonella* infections,[35] and avoiding travel to areas with endemic fungal infections when climatic conditions favor inhalation of *Histoplasma capsulatum* or *Coccidioides immitis*.[36,37]

Maintenance Therapy

In addition to efficient management of chemoprophylaxis and reducing risk of exposure, a third component of preventive therapy is maintenance therapy to prevent relapse after successful treatment of an acute opportunistic infection. PCP, toxoplasmosis, invasive fungal infections, CMV retinitis, and disseminated MAC infection all require lifelong therapy to prevent relapse in HIV-1 infected persons. This is addressed in a later chapter.

Clearly, the most effective method of preventing opportunistic infections requires identification and treatment of HIV-1 infected individuals with effective early antiretroviral therapy to prevent the loss of immune competence. Effective antiretroviral therapy initiated later in the course of infection, after the CD4$^+$ lymphocyte count falls below 200/mm^3, often results in an increase of these cells to above this level. It is not known if prophylaxis to prevent opportunistic infections such as PCP or disseminated MAC can be safely discontinued in individuals who have had a good response to antiviral therapy. Preliminary evidence suggests that the increased number of CD4$^+$ lymphocytes do not reflect a normal distribution of these cells. A permanent loss of the clones of cells capable of controlling specific latent infections or preventing infection from exogenous exposure to specific opportunistic pathogens may have occurred. Until evidence from controlled studies is available to answer this question, continuation of prophylactic regimens appears advisable.

References

1.   Fischl MA, Dikinson GM, LaVore L: Safety and efficacy of sulfamethoxazole and trimethoprim chemoprophylaxis for *Pneumocystis carinii* pneumonia in AIDS. *JAMA* 1988;259:1185-1189.

2.   Leoung GS, Feigal DW, Montgomery AB, et al: Aerosolized pentamidine for prophylaxis against *Pneumocystis carinii* pneumonia. *N Engl J Med* 1990;323:769-775.

3.   Phair JP, Muñoz A, Detels R: The risk of *Pneumocystis carinii* pneumonia among men infected with human immunodeficiency virus type-1. *N Engl J Med* 1990;322:161-165.

4.   Kirby AJ, Muñoz A, Detels R, et al: Thrush and fever as measures of immunocompetence in HIV-1 infected men. *J Acquir Immune Defic Syndr* 1994;7:1242-1249.

5.   Centers for Disease Control: Guidelines for prophylaxis against *Pneumocystis carinii* pneumonia for persons infected with human immunodeficiency virus. *MMWR* 1989;38(suppl 5):1-9.

6.   Centers for Disease Control: Recommendation for prophylaxis against *Pneumocystis carinii* pneumonia for adults and adolescents infected with human immunodeficiency virus. *MMWR* 1992;41 (RR-4):1-11.

7.   Centers for Disease Control: Guidelines for prophylaxis against *Pneumocystis carinii* pneumonia for children infected with human immunodeficiency virus. *MMWR* 1991;40(RR-2):1-13.

8.   Kaplan JE, Masur H, Holmes KK, eds: Prevention of opportunistic infections in persons infected with human immunodeficiency virus. *Clin Infect Dis* 1995;21(suppl 1):S1-S141.

9.   Centers for Disease Control and Prevention: 1997 USPHS/IDSA guidelines for the prevention of opportunistic infections in persons infected with human immunodeficiency virus. *MMWR* 1997;46:1-46.

10.   Hoover DR, Saah AJ, Bacellar H, et al: Clinical manifestations of AIDS in the era of pneumocystis prophylaxis. Multicenter AIDS Cohort Study. *N Engl J Med* 1993;329:1922-1926.

11.   Osmond D, Charlebois E, Lang W, et al: Changes in AIDS survival time in two San Francisco cohorts of homosexual men 1983 to 1993. *JAMA* 1994;271:1083-1087.

12.   Bozzette SA, Finkelstein DM, Spector SA, et al: A randomized trial of three antipneumocystis agents in patients with advanced human immunodeficiency virus infection. *N Engl J Med* 1995;332:693-699.

13.   Sha B, Benson C, Deutsche T, et al: *Pneumocystis carinii* choroiditis in patients with AIDS; clinical features, response to therapy and outcome. *J Acquir Immune Defic Syndr* 1992;5:1051-1058.

14.   Saah A, Hoover DR, Peng Y, et al: Predictors for failure of *Pneumocystis carinii* pneumonia prophylaxis. *JAMA* 1995;273:1197-1202.

15.   Richards FO, Kovacs JA, Luft BJ: Preventing toxoplasmic encephalitis in persons infected with human immunodeficiency virus. *Clin Infect Dis* 1995;2(suppl 1):S49-S56.

16.   Carr A, Tindall B, Brew BJ, et al: Low dose trimethoprim-sulfamethoxazole prophylaxis for toxoplasmic encephalitis in patients with AIDS. *Ann Intern Med* 1992;117:106-111.

17. Leport C, Chenc G, Morlat P, et al: Pyrimethamine for primary prophylaxis of toxoplasmic encephalitis in patients with human immunodeficiency virus infection: a double-blind randomized trial. *J Infect Dis* 1996;173:91-97.

18. Kandree MA: High prevalence of trimethoprim-sulfamethoxazole (TMP/SMX) resistant *Streptococcus pneumoniae* sulfamethoxazole in HIV-infected patients on TMP/SMX for pneumocystis prophylaxis: therapeutic implications. XI International Conference of AIDS, Vancouver, BC, July 1996, Abstract Tu.B.182.

19. Benson CA, Cohen DL, Williams P, et al: A phase III prospective, randomized, double-blind study of the safety and efficacy of clarithromycin vs. rifabutin vs. clarithromycin plus rifabutin for prevention of MAC in HIV+ patients with CD4 counts <100 cells/mL. Third Conference on Retroviruses and Opportunistic Infections. Washington, DC. January 1996, Abstract 204.

20. Havlir DV, Duke MP, Sattler FR, et al: Prophylaxis against disseminated *Mycobacterium avium* complex with weekly azithromycin, daily rifabutin or both. *N Engl J Med* 1996;335;392-398.

21. Nightingale SD, Cameron DW, Gordon FM, et al: Two controlled trials of rifabutin prophylaxis against *Mycobacterium avium* complex infection in AIDS. *N Engl J Med* 1993;329:828-833.

22. Moore RD, Chaisson RE: Survival analysis of two controlled trials of rifabutin prophylaxis against *Mycobacterium avium* complex in AIDS. *AIDS* 1995;9:1337-1342.

23. Masur H: Recommendation on prophylaxis and therapy for disseminated *Mycobacterium avium* complex disease in patients infected with human immunodeficiency virus. *N Engl J Med* 1993;329:898-904.

24. Abbott Pharmaceuticals: Norvir package insert.

25. Powderly WG, Finkelstein OM, Fineberg J: A randomized trial comparing fluconazole with clotrimazole troches for the prevention of fungal infections in patients with advanced human immunodeficiency virus infection. *N Engl J Med* 1995;332:700-705.

26. Reef SE, Mayer KH: Opportunistic *Candida* infections in patients infected with human immunodeficiency virus; prevention issues and priorities. *Clin Infect Dis* 1995;21(suppl 1):S99-S102.

26. Pertel P, Hirschtick R, Phair JP, et al: Risk of developing CMV retinitis in persons infected with the human immunodeficiency virus. *J Acquir Immune Defic Syndr* 1992;5:1069-1974.

27. Spector SA, McKinley GG, Lalezari JP, et al: Oral ganciclovir for the prevention of cytomegalovirus disease in persons with AIDS. *N Engl J Med* 1996;334:1491-1497.

28. Bosgart C, Craig C, Hillman D, et al: Final results from a randomized placebo-controlled trial of the safety and efficacy of oral ganciclovir for prophylaxis of CMV retinal and gastrointestinal mucosa. XI International Conference on AIDS, Vancouver, BC, July 1996, Abstract LB-10.

29. Feinberg J, Cooper D, Horowitz S, et al: Phase III international study of valacyclovir for cytomegalovirus prophylaxis in patients with advanced HIV infection. XI International Conference on AIDS, Vancouver, BC, July 1996, Abstract Th.B.300.

30. Spector SA, Pilcher M, Larry P, et al: PCR of plasma for cytomegalovirus DNA identifies HIV-infected persons most likely to benefit from oral ganciclovir prophylaxis. XI International Conference on AIDS, Vancouver, BC, July 1996, Abstract Th.B.302.

31. Griffith PD, Feinberg J: Detection of cytomegalovirus in samples from patients enrolled in ACTG 204. Third Conference on Retroviruses and Opportunistic Infection, Washington, DC, January 1996, Abstract 10.

32. Hoover DR, Graham NM, Bacellar H, et al: An epidemiologic analysis of *Mycobacterium avium* complex disease in homosexual men infected with human immunodeficiency virus type-1. *Clin Infect Dis* 1995;20:250-258.

33. Castro KG: Tuberculosis as an opportunistic disease in persons infected with human immunodeficiency virus. *Clin Infect Dis* 1995;21(suppl 1):S66-S71.

34. Juranels DD: Cryptosporidiosis: sources of infection and guidelines for prevention. *Clin Infect Dis* 1995;21(suppl 1):S57-S61.

35. Regnery RC, Childs JE, Koehler JE: Infections associated with *Bartonella* species in persons infected with human immunodeficiency virus. *Clin Infect Dis* 1995;21(suppl 1):S94-S98.

36. Hajjeh RA: Disseminated histoplasmosis in persons infected with human immunodeficiency virus. *Clin Infect Dis* 1995;21 (suppl 1): S108-S110.

37. McNeil MM, Ampel NM: Opportunistic coccidioidomycosis in patients infected with human immunodeficiency virus: prevention issue and priorities. *Clin Infect Dis* 1995;21(suppl 1):S111-S113.

Chapter 7

Treatment of Opportunistic Infections of HIV Disease

Candidiasis

The pseudomembranous form of oral or vaginal candidiasis is one of the more common clinical manifestations of HIV-1 disease. The presence of this mucocutaneous form of candidiasis suggests the presence of a significant immunologic deficiency and is predictive of the rapid development of full-blown clinical AIDS in the HIV-1 seropositive patient.[1] The most common clinical presentation is that of removable white plaques located on an erythematous base of any mucosal surface. Without the easily removable white plaques, the erythematous form is less common and often overlooked or misdiagnosed. Angular cheilitis is a form of *Candida* infection that produces cracks, fissures, and erythema at the corners of the mouth.[2,3]

Candidiasis is often diagnosed after clinical observation and response to specific antifungal therapy. The diagnosis is confirmed either with potassium hydroxide preparation of a smear taken directly from the lesion, or with a culture that may determine the species involved and the susceptibility to specific antifungal agents.

A more extensive form of candidiasis is esophagitis, a formal AIDS-defining condition. Symptoms associated with esophageal candidiasis typically include dysphagia, odynophagia, and retrosternal pain. Most of these patients will have concomitant oral candidiasis.[4] The diagnosis of esophageal candidiasis can be clinical and can include a positive response to therapy. Characteristic endoscopic findings with tissue-invading pseudomycelia seen in the biopsy can be used to confirm the diagnosis. A fungal culture or brush cytology of suspicious esophageal lesions strongly suggests this diagnosis when seen in the presence of the compatible clinical syndrome. A barium contrast radiograph may suggest, but not document, the diagnosis.

Treatment of the various forms of candidiasis is relatively routine in most instances and ranges from local to systemic therapies, both oral and parenteral. The type of therapy depends on the site and severity of the infection, as well as on the susceptibility of the organism involved (Table 1). Very advanced disease and extensive prior antifungal therapy may increase the likelihood of resistance to certain agents.

Coccidioidomycosis

Coccidioidomycosis is caused by the fungal organism *Coccidioides immitis*, which is endemic to the southwestern United States, northern Mexico, and portions of Central America. Infection occurs after inhalation of infectious mycelial forms. In Arizona, coccidioidomycosis is the third most common AIDS-defining infection and typically occurs in patients with less than 250 CD4$^+$ cells/mm^3 and negative spherulin skin tests.[5,6]

The clinical presentation of coccidioidal infection ranges from a positive serologic skin test to life-threatening pneumonitis or meningitis. Diffuse pulmonary disease is common and may mimic other opportunistic diseases such as *Pneumocystis carinii* pneumonia or miliary tuberculosis. Cutaneous lesions may occur with or without other disease manifestations. Coccidioidal meningitis is characterized by high cerebral leukocyte counts in the spinal fluid and hypoglycorrhachia.

Coccidioidomycosis is diagnosed using a culture of the organism from the infected clinical site. Nearly all patients have a positive serologic titer for *C immitis* at diagnosis.

Table 1: Treatment of Candidiasis

Disease/location	Preferred treatment
oral	fluconazole 50-100 mg PO x 7-14 days
cheilitis	clotrimazole 2% cream or ketoconazole cream applied locally b.i.d. until cleared
esophagitis	fluconazole 200 mg PO x 1 dose, then 100 mg daily for 7-14 days or until symptoms resolve (may require chronic maintenance therapy)
vaginitis	(1) clotrimazole 100 mg vaginal suppositories qhs for 3 nights, or
	(2) fluconazole 100-200 mg PO daily for 3 days, or
	(3) miconazole 200 mg vaginal suppositories qhs for 3 nights, or
	(4) terconazole 80 mg vaginal suppositories qhs for 3 nights, or
	(5) itraconazole 200 mg PO daily for 3 days

Treatment is with amphotericin B (Fungizone®), especially for patients with diffuse pulmonary disease. Chronic maintenance therapy with azole antifungal agents is warranted. As with other serious systemic fungal infections, the infection should be stabilized and a minimum of 500 to 1000 mg amphotericin B administered before switching to oral azole treatment. There is evidence that oral fluconazole may be the preferred treatment for meningitis (Table 2). Fluconazole

Alternative therapies

(1) amphotericin B 20 mg IV daily or 50 mg IV 2-3 x week until signs and symptoms resolve for azole-resistant and severe disease only

(2) clotrimazole 10 mg troches 5 x daily for 7-14 days

(3) ketoconazole 200 mg PO x 7-14 days

(4) itraconazole oral solution 200 mg PO q.d. for 7-14 days

(5) nystatin solution or pastilles 100,000-500,000 units; swish and swallow or dissolve in mouth for 1-2 weeks

(1) amphotericin B 20 mg IV daily or 50 mg IV 2-3 x week until symptoms resolve (for azole-resistant candidiasis and severe disease only)

(2) itraconazole oral solution 200 mg PO q.d. for 1-3 weeks

(3) ketoconazole 200 mg PO daily for 1-2 weeks

(Diflucan®) and itraconazole (Sporanox®) appear to be effective in treating coccidioidomycosis, whereas ketoconazole does not.

Cryptococcosis

Cryptococcosis refers to the systemic fungal disease caused by *Cryptococcus neoformans*. Disease can occur in patients with underlying immune deficiencies such as lymphoma and

Table 2: Treatment of Coccidioidomycosis

Site of infection	Preferred treatment	Alternate treatment
meningitis	fluconazole 400 mg daily, increase to 800 mg if no response	amphotericin B 0.1-0.3 mg intrathecally daily if no response to fluconazole
pulmonary or fungemia	amphotericin B 0.6-1.2 mg/kg daily until symptoms resolve, then fluconazole 400 mg PO daily	(1) fluconazole 400 mg PO daily, or (2) itraconazole 200 mg PO b.i.d.
other	(1) fluconazole 400 mg PO daily, or (2) itraconazole 200 mg PO b.i.d.	

diabetes, and in those who receive immunosuppressive therapies, such as corticosteroids. In patients with AIDS, cryptococcosis is the fourth most common AIDS-defining condition, occurring in 6% to 10% in this population.[7] The incidence of cryptococcal disease may actually be declining.[8]

Infection occurs after inhalation of the organism. Surprisingly, most clinical disease is extrapulmonary and the central nervous system is the site most commonly involved. The onset of symptoms is insidious, and may be present for weeks before the diagnosis is confirmed. Headache, fever, and malaise are the most common symptoms of meningitis. Less than one third have nuchal rigidity or focal neurologic signs.[9] Extral neural disease is present in 20% to 60% of cases; pulmonary involvement occurs in 20% to 30%.

The diagnosis of cryptococcal disease is confirmed with a positive culture from the infected site. The serum and cerebral spinal fluid cryptococcal antigen test is usually positive. A lumbar puncture is recommended for patients with meningitis to confirm the diagnosis and for therapeutic reasons. This proce

Table 3: Treatment of Cryptococcosis

	Preferred treatment	Alternative treatment
systemic disease	amphotericin B 0.7 mg/kg IV daily until patient is afebrile and symptoms resolve plus flucytosine (5-FC) 25-37.5 mg/kg PO every 6 h while taking amphotericin B. Follow this with fluconazole 400 mg PO daily for 10 weeks, then 200 mg PO daily indefinitely	fluconazole 400 mg PO daily for 12 weeks, then 200 mg PO daily indefinitely

dure should be performed after an imaging scan of the brain to ensure that a space-occupying mass lesion, such as a lymphoma or toxoplasmic abscess, is not present. In contrast to patients without AIDS, the spinal fluid may have few abnormalities other than high opening pressure (>200 mm H_2O) and a positive India ink preparation and cryptococcal antigen. Low leukocyte count (<20 cells/mm^3), altered mental status, and a cerebral fluid cryptococcal antigen titer greater than or equal to 1:1024 are all markers of severe disease that require aggressive therapy.

The initial treatment of acute cryptococcal meningitis is with amphotericin B plus flucytosine (Ancobon®). In the absence of obstructive hydrocephalus, repeat lumbar punctures with removal of 10 mm^3 to 20 mm^3 of spinal fluid is recommended for patients with an elevated opening pressure greater than 200 mm H_2O. Therapy is indefinite, although maintenance doses can be lowered (Table 3).

Cryptosporidiosis

One of the more common causes of AIDS-associated diarrhea is infection with the protozoan *Cryptosporidium parvum*. Typical symptoms include watery diarrhea, weight loss, abdominal pain, nausea, and vomiting. Fever is unusual. The large or small bowel may be involved and, to a lesser extent, the hepatobiliary tree. The diagnosis can usually be made by examination of the stool for the presence of the acid-fast staining cysts. In some instances, an intestinal biopsy will be required to confirm the diagnosis.

Treatment of cryptosporidiosis is unsatisfactory from an antimicrobial perspective. At present, nonspecific antidiarrheal agents play a prominent role in relieving the symptoms of this disease.

Histoplasmosis

Histoplasmosis is caused by the fungus *Histoplasma capsulatum*. The disease is endemic in the central and southern regions of the United States, parts of Canada, Mexico, and Central and South America. In some areas of the United States, such as Indiana, histoplasmosis is the second or third most common AIDS-defining infection.[11] Infection occurs after inhalation of arthroconidia, which rapidly convert to the yeast phase in the body and disseminate to target organs. In the normal host, clinical disease is unusual. In AIDS, clinical disease is either acute or caused by reactivation of latent infection.

As with the other opportunistic infections, histoplasmosis occurs late in the AIDS disease process. The median CD4$^+$ count at the time of diagnosis is typically below 50 cells/mm^3.[12] Fever, weight loss, and constitutional symptoms are common in most patients. Respiratory complaints are observed in 50% to 60%, hepatosplenomegaly in 20% to 40%, neurologic signs and symptoms in 20%, lymphadenopathy in 20%, and skin and mucosal involvement in 2% to 5%.[13]

The diagnosis of histoplasmosis is confirmed with a culture from an infected site. This may take 2 to 3 weeks. Histopathologic identification can be accomplished in about 50% of cases. Standard serologic assays are generally not helpful; however, a *Histoplasma* antigen test of urine or serum is sensitive and highly specific for active disease. Serum *Histoplasma* antigen titers typically fall by 2 units after successful therapy.[14]

Table 4: Treatment of Histoplasmosis

	Preferred treatment	Alternative treatement
severe disease: meningeal, septic	amphotericin B 50 mg IV daily for total of 10-15 mg/kg, then itraconazole 200 mg PO b.i.d. indefinitely	itraconazole 200 mg t.i.d. x 3 days then b.i.d. indefinitely
less severe disease	itraconazole 200 mg PO t.i.d. x 3 days then b.i.d.	

Initial treatment of histoplasmosis is with amphotericin B, followed by indefinite use of itraconazole. In less severe disease, treatment with itraconazole alone may be sufficient (Table 4).[15]

Microsporidiosis

Microsporidiosis refers to the protozoan disease that is common in patients with refractory diarrhea. At least two species, *Enterocytozoon bienusi* and *Encephalitozoon cuniculi*, have been implicated in human disease. Typically, patients have watery diarrhea, weight loss, and abdominal pain. Fever and anorexia are uncommon. Stool examination is remarkable for no other known pathogens and few leukocytes, if any.

The diagnosis of microsporidiosis is difficult. The most reliable diagnostic test is examination of a small bowel biopsy specimen by electron microscopy. Treatment is also difficult, although successful responses with albendazole and atovaquone (Mepron®) have been reported (Table 5).[16,17]

Mycobacterium avium Complex Disease

Dissemination of the bacterium *Mycobacterium avium* is one of the more important AIDS-defining infections. Its incidence is increasing in the United States. Disease caused by *Mycobacterium avium* is associated with late-stage

Table 5: Treatment of Microsporidiosis

Preferred treatment
albendazole, 400-800 mg b.i.d.
(especially *E cuniculi*)

Alternative
atovaquone suspension, 750 mg t.i.d.

AIDS and shortened survival.[18] *Mycobacterium avium* is ubiquitous in soil and water, and the source of infection in humans may be through either the gastrointestinal tract or the lungs.[19]

Mycobacterium avium complex disseminates widely throughout the body. Nearly all patients with the disease will have positive blood cultures. Colonization without disease may occur in respiratory secretions, stool, and urine; however, the associated organ systems can become infected as well. Histopathology of infected tissues typically reveals large numbers of acid-fast staining organisms within macrophages and few, if any, poorly formed granulomas.

Clinically, most patients with MAC have fever, weight loss, and malaise. Anemia, diarrhea, and obstructive jaundice may be present, depending on the severity and type of organ involvement. Diagnosis is made with culture of blood or other tissue, but the clinical relevance of sputum or stool culture is controversial. In one study, two thirds of patients with negative blood cultures but positive stool or sputum cultures for MAC subsequently developed disseminated MAC.[20]

Treatment of MAC (Table 6) involves at least two drugs—clarithromycin (Biaxin®) and ethambutol (Myambutol®). High doses of clarithromycin (2 g per day) do not increase efficacy rates.[21] Clofazimine (Lamprene®) adds no efficacy and may be associated with higher mortality.[22] Other drugs that have been used to treat MAC include azithromycin (Zithromax®) , which may be cross-resistant with clarithromycin, rifabutin (Mycobutin®), and ciprofloxacin (Cipro®).

Table 6: Treatment of *Mycobacterium avium* Complex Disease

Preferred treatment	Alternate treatment
clarithromycin 500 mg PO b.i.d. plus	(1) azithromycin 500-600 mg PO daily can be substituted for clarithromycin
ethambutol 15-25 mg/kg PO daily	(2) rifabutin 450-600 mg PO daily or
	(3) ciprofloxacin 750 mg PO q.d. or b.i.d. can be substituted or added to the other regimens

Mycobacterium tuberculosis

Tuberculosis has become an important complication of AIDS. Because of the specific immunologic deficiency associated with HIV-1 infection, it increases the risk of developing clinical tuberculosis. Moreover, HIV-1 infection complicates factors such as homelessness, incarceration, substance abuse, and poor socioeconomic conditions that are common to many patients with HIV.[23] The importance of the interaction between HIV-1 infection and tuberculosis can be summarized by the following factors: the prevalence of tuberculosis is high in certain HIV-1 infected groups; tuberculosis is probably the only HIV-1 related infection that is transmitted person-to-person, whether or not the exposed person is infected with HIV-1; despite HIV-1 infection, tuberculosis can be cured if diagnosed promptly and treated appropriately; tuberculosis can be prevented in HIV-1 infected populations by prophylaxis and sound and reasonable public health measures; and tuberculosis may accelerate the course of HIV.[24]

The overall median HIV-1 seropositivity rate among American patients with suspected or proven tuberculosis who attended 14 urban tuberculosis clinics was reported to be 3.4%; however, the rates varied from 0% to 46%, with the highest rate occurring in New York City.[25] In developing countries, a substantial rate of HIV-1 infection occurs among those with tuberculosis, which makes it the most common serious infection in AIDS in certain areas, such as sub-Saharan Africa.

Tuberculosis can develop after primary exposure to *M tuberculosis,* or it can reactivate from latent infection. Both of these routes of acquisition are important to individuals infected with HIV-1. Tuberculosis tends to occur relatively early in the course of HIV-1 infection. For example, in one study, the median $CD4^+$ count at the time of diagnosis was 354 cells/mm^3.[26] Tuberculosis tends to progress more rapidly in persons with HIV-1, who are more likely to be anergic or have a blunted skin-test response to the tuberculin-purified protein derivative. Because of this, a positive skin-test response in an HIV-1 infected person is defined as a reaction of greater than or equal to 5 mm induration.[27]

The clinical manifestations of tuberculosis in patients with HIV-1 infection vary widely and depend mainly on the stage of immunosuppression of the individual patient. In general, as the HIV-1 disease progresses, tuberculosis is more likely to present as a disseminated disease, with unusual pulmonary manifestations and extrapulmonary involvement that includes lymph nodes, central nervous system, bone, and blood.[28] The radiographic presentation of patients with tuberculosis and HIV-1 infection range from the typical cavitary upper lobe disease to that of a higher frequency of adenopathy and lower lobe infiltration with less cavitation.

The diagnosis of tuberculosis relies on culture of infected sputum or tissue. The use of a polymerase chain reaction for identification of *M tuberculosis* may result in a more rapid diagnosis, but it is not more sensitive than culture and its clinical use has yet to be fully established.[29]

Treatment of tuberculosis in patients with HIV-1 infection is generally successful if the appropriate therapy is promptly initiated and the patient is compliant. Current successful regi-

Table 7: Treatment of Tuberculosis

Preferred treatment*

isoniazid 300 mg
PO daily, plus

pyridoxine 50 mg
PO daily, plus

rifampin 600 mg
PO daily (450 mg for
persons <50 kg), plus

pyrazinamide 20-30 mg/kg
PO daily, plus

ethambutol 15 mg/kg PO daily

*after 2 months, the pyrazinamide and ethambutol can be discontinued;
the isoniazid, pyridoxine, and rifampin should be continued for at least
6 months

mens include isoniazid and rifampin. During the first 2 months
of therapy, pyrazinamide and ethambutol should also be administered. Therapy should be directly observed for those patients with a suspected compliance problem (Table 7).

Disease caused by multidrug-resistant (MDR) organisms
poses difficult challenges in areas with a high prevalence of
drug resistance to one or more of the commonly used antitu-
berculous agents. Prompt recognition and treatment of resistant organisms are critical although very difficult. Therapy
must be tailored according to the known or suspected resistance patterns in the community. At least two agents known
to be sensitive to the isolate being treated should be used.
Treatment should continue for 24 months at most after con-
version to negative (Table 8).[30]

Pneumocystosis

Pneumocystosis refers to disease caused by the organism
Pneumocystis carinii. Formerly classified as a protozoan, it
is now thought that *P carinii* is more like fungi. Recent classification places it among the ascomycetes.[31] Infection is
thought to follow inhalation of infectious particles. By the

Table 8: Potential Regimens for Patients With Tuberculosis With Various Patterns of Drug Resistance

Resistance	Suggested Regimen
isoniazid, streptomycin, and pyrazinamide	rifampin pyrazinamide ethambutol amikacin[a]
isoniazid and ethambutol (±streptomycin)	rifampin pyrazinamide ofloxacin or ciprofloxacin amikacin[a]
isoniazid and rifampin (±streptomycin)	pyrazinamide ethambutol ofloxacin or ciprofloxacin amikacin[a]
isoniazid, rifampin, and ethambutol (±streptomycin)	pyrazinamide ofloxacin or ciprofloxacin amikacin[a] plus 2 from list of potential agents[b]
isoniazid, rifampin, and pyrazinamide (±streptomycin)	ethambutol ofloxacin or ciprofloxacin amikacin[a] plus 2 from list of potential agents[b]
isoniazid, rifampin, pyrazinamide, and ethambutol (±streptomycin)	ofloxacin or ciprofloxacin plus 3 from list of potential agents[b] amikacin[a]

[a] If there is resistance to amikacin, kanamycin, and streptomycin, capreomycin is a good alternative. Injectable agents are usually continued for 4 to 6 months if toxicity does not intervene. All the injectable drugs are given daily (or 2 or 3 times weekly) and may be administered intravenously or intramuscularly.

Duration of Therapy	Comments
6 to 9 months	Anticipate 100% response rate and 5% relapse rate
6 to 12 months to above regimen	Efficacy should be comparable
18 to 24 months	Consider surgery
24 months after conversion	Consider surgery
24 months after conversion	Consider surgery
24 months after conversion	Surgery, if possible

[b] Potential agents from which to choose: ethionamide, cycloserine, or aminosalicylic acid. Others that are potentially useful but of unproven utility include clofazimine and amoxicillin/clavulanate. Clarithromycin, azithromycin, and ritabutin are unlikely to be active.

Table 9a: Treatment of Mild to Moderate *Pneumocystis carinii* Pneumonia

Treatment regimen	Dosages
trimethoprim-sulfamethoxazole	2 DS tablets PO t.i.d.
trimethoprim-dapsone	trimethoprim 100 mg PO t.i.d., plus dapsone 100 mg PO daily
clindamycin-primaquine	clindamycin 600 mg PO t.i.d., plus primaquine 30 mg PO daily
atovaquone	750 mg suspension PO t.i.d.
pentamidine isoethionate	3 mg/kg IV daily
trimetrexate-leucovorin	trimetrexate 45 mg/m^2 IV daily, plus leucovorin 20 mg/m^2 PO q.i.d. during treatment and for 3 days after completion

Note: All treatment should be for 21 days.

age of 4 years, most humans have developed an antibody response to specific *P carinii* antigens. Initial disease in adults, although originally thought to be a reactivation of latent disease, is likely to be from acute exposure to the organism.[32] Relapse after pneumonia may be from incompletely eradicated organisms from the lung, but even this is not certain.[33] At this point, it is not known whether person-to-person transmission of *P carinii* is clinically relevant.

The usual clinical presentation of pneumocystosis in the adult is a pulmonary process, referred to as *Pneumocystis carinii* pneumonia (PCP). Infrequently, other organ systems may become infected, particularly when aerosolized forms of prophylaxis are administered for prolonged periods. Pneumocystosis usually occurs late in the course of HIV-1 disease and is the most common AIDS-defining opportunis-

Adverse events

rash, fever, nausea, vomiting, neutropenia, elevated liver transaminases

rash, fever, nausea, vomiting, neutropenia, elevated liver transaminases; hemolytic anemia (especially in G6PD-deficient patients), methemoglobinemia

rash, nausea, vomiting, diarrhea; hemolytic anemia (especially G6PD-deficient patients), methemoglobinemia

rash, nausea, vomiting, diarrhea, unusual taste and color; may not be absorbed in persons with diarrhea

nephrotoxicity, nausea, vomiting, hypotension, pancreatitis, hypoglycemia

neutropenia, thrombocytopenia, anemia, rash, fever, liver transaminase elevation

tic infection. Risk factors for pneumocystosis include CD4$^+$ cell count less than 200 cells/mm^3, oral thrush, and unexplained fever.[34] The incidence of PCP has declined in recent years, primarily because of the widespread use of effective prophylactic therapies administered to individuals at risk.

The clinical presentation of PCP commonly starts with fever and slowly progressive dyspnea with nonproductive cough. These symptoms will gradually progress, usually over several weeks, and can become severe. Physical examination is remarkable for fever and tachypnea. Auscultation of the lungs is often normal, especially early in the course of the disease. Laboratory abnormalities are nonspecific. The lactate dehydrogenase (LDH) can be elevated; however, this is a nonspecific finding. The chest radiograph is typically a diffuse, interstitial infiltrate. Pneumatoceles may be present and

Table 9b: Treatment of Moderate to Severe *Pneumocystis carinii* Pneumonia

Treatment	Dosages	Side effects
trimethoprim-sulfamethoxazole	15-20 mg/kg (trimethoprim component) IV divided every 6 h	see Table 9a
clindamycin-primaquine	clindamycin 900 mg IV q 8 h, plus primaquine 30 mg PO daily	see Table 9a
pentamidine	3-4 mg/kg IV daily	see Table 9a
trimetrexate-leucovorin	trimetrexate 45 mg/m² IV daily, plus leucovorin 20 mg/m² PO or IV q 6 h for the course of therapy and for 3 days after completion of trimetrexate	see Table 9a
prednisone (in addition to one of the above therapies)	40 mg PO b.i.d. x first 5 days, then 40 mg PO q.d. x next 5 days, then 20 mg PO q.d. for the remaining 11 days of therapy	psychosis, irritability, may accelerate non-PCP infection processes and Kaposi's sarcoma

Note: All treatment should be for 21 days.

pneumothorax may occur. In some series, early chest radiographs are completely normal.

Pneumocystis carinii pneumonia is diagnosed by identification of characteristic *P carinii* cysts from an induced sputum or bronchial lavage specimen in a patient with a compatible syndrome. If the sputum induction is negative, a single-breath diffusing capacity for carbon monoxide or a high-resolution computed tomograph (CT) of the chest may be helpful in evaluating a patient with suspected disease.

Table 10a: Preferred Treatment of Toxoplasmosis

Preferred treatment	Dosage	Side effects
pyrimethamine, plus	200 mg PO loading dose, then 50-75 mg PO daily for 3-6 weeks, then 25-50 mg PO daily	seizures, rash, atrophic glossitis, vomiting, agranulocytosis, and anemia; must be taken with leucovorin 10-20 mg PO daily
sulfadiazine, or	500-1000 mg PO q.i.d.	rash, nausea, vomiting, fever, toxic nephrosis, anemia, agranulocytosis
clindamycin	900 mg IV q 8 h or 600 mg PO q 6 h for 3-6 weeks, then 300-450 mg PO q 6-12 h daily	rash, diarrhea, nausea, vomiting

Treatment of PCP depends on the severity of the disease. For mild to moderate disease (partial oxygen pressure [PO_2] >70 mm Hg or an alveolar-arterial difference <35 mm Hg), four oral regimens are recommended (Table 9a). For more severe disease, four parenteral regimens are recommended in conjunction with adjuvant corticosteroid therapy (Table 9b). When administered with specific anti-PCP treatment, corticosteroids—either oral prednisone or intravenous methylprednisolone—have been clearly shown to reduce the likelihood of death, respiratory failure, or deterioration of oxygenation in patients with moderate to severe PCP.[35]

Trimethoprim-sulfamethoxazole (TMP-SMX) remains the drug of choice for treatment of all cases of PCP. The problem has been high intolerance rates, the exact mechanism of which has yet to be determined. Approximately one

Table 10b: Alternate Treatment of Toxoplasmosis

Alternate treatment	Dosage	Side effects
pyrimethamine, plus	200 mg PO loading dose, then 50-75 mg PO daily for 3-6 weeks, then 25-50 mg PO daily	see Table 10a
atovaquone, or	750 mg suspension PO q 6 h	rash, nausea, vomiting, diarrhea, unusual taste and color; may not be absorbed if diarrhea present
azithromycin, or	1200-1500 mg PO daily	diarrhea, nausea, abdominal pain
dapsone, or	100 mg PO daily	hemolytic anemia (especially G6PD-deficient patients), methemoglobinemia, rash, nausea, vomiting
clarithromycin	1000 mg PO b.i.d.	nausea, vomiting, diarrhea, headache, abnormal taste; terfenadine contraindicated

third of patients cannot complete a treatment course of TMP-SMX because of intolerance or toxicity.[36]

Toxoplasmosis

Toxoplasmosis refers to the disease caused by the protozoan organism *Toxoplasma gondii*. People are exposed to *T gondii* primarily by ingestion of undercooked meat contaminated with oocysts or by direct contact with cat feces. In persons with AIDS, toxoplasmosis is a result of disease activation of latent infection. The most common presentation is encephalitis, although, less commonly, ocular, lung, heart, and other sites may become infected. Infection seroprevalence rates in the United States range from 8% to 16% in urban areas, but are much higher in developing nations. As many as 47% of seropositive patients with advanced AIDS will develop toxoplasmic encephalitis.[37]

The typical clinical presentation of toxoplasmic encephalitis is the subacute onset of focal neurologic abnormalities. Altered mental status, seizures, and coma may also be presenting signs. The diagnosis of toxoplasmosis is based on a compatible clinical history and examination of a patient with a positive *Toxoplasma* serology and with imaging studies of the brain that reveal multiple ring-enhancing lesions. The most sensitive imaging study is the magnetic resonance (MR) scan of the brain; however, double-contrast CT is usually helpful and generally more readily available.[38] Although confirmatory, biopsy of the suspected brain lesion is infrequently indicated unless there is no response to empiric treatment or only a single lesion is observed on MR scan.

Treatment of acute toxoplasmosis is with pyrimethamine plus sulfadiazine (Microsulfon®) or clindamycin (Cleocin®) (Table 10a). Patients who cannot tolerate sulfadiazine or clindamycin can be given atovaquone, azithromycin, clarithromycin, or dapsone as substitutes (Table 10b). A few studies have suggested that TMP-SMX may be effective in treating acute disease. However, efficacy rates are inferior to the other standard regimens.[39]

References

1. Phair JP, Munoz A, Detels R, et al: The risk of *Pneumocystis carinii* pneumonia among men infected with human immunodeficiency type 1. *N Engl J Med* 1990;322:161-165.

2. Dodd CL, Greenspan D, Katz MH, et al: Oral candidiasis in HIV infection: pseudomembranous and erythematous candidiasis show similar rates of progression to AIDS. *AIDS* 1991;5:1339-1343.

3. Greenspan JS, Barr CE, Sciubba JJ, et al: Oral manifestations of HIV infection: definitions, diagnostic criteria and principles of therapy. *Oral Surg Oral Med Oral Pathol* 1992;73:142-144.

4. Laine L, Dretler RH, Conteas CN, et al: Fluconazole compared with ketoconazole for the treatment of *Candida* esophagitis in AIDS. *Ann Intern Med* 1992;117:655-660.

5. Fish DG, Ampel NM, Galgiani JN, et al: Coccidioidomycosis during human immunodeficiency virus infection: a review of 77 patients. *Medicine* 1990;69:384-391.

6. Galgiani JN, Ampel NM: Coccidioidomycosis in human immunodeficiency virus-infected patients. *J Infect Dis* 1990;162:1165-1169.

7. Clark RA, Greer D, Atkinson W, et al: Spectrum of *Cryptococcus neoformans* in 68 patients infected with human immunodeficiency virus. *Rev Infect Dis* 1990;12:768-777.

8. Moore RD, Chaisson RE: Natural history of opportunistic disease in an HIV-infected urban clinical cohort. *Ann Intern Med* 1996;124:633-642.

9. Chuck SL, Sande MA: Infections with *Cryptococcus neoformans* in the acquired immunodeficiency syndrome. *N Engl J Med* 1989; 321:794-799.

10. Van der Horst CM, Saag MS, Cloud GA, et al: Treatment of cryptococcal meningitis associated with the acquired immunodeficiency syndrome. *N Engl J Med* 1997;337:15-21.

11. Sarosi GA, Johnson PC: Disseminated histoplasmosis in patients with human immunodeficiency virus. *Clin Infect Dis* 1992; 14:S60-S67.

12. Wheat LJ, Connolly-Stringfield P, Baker RL, et al: Disseminated histoplasmosis in the acquired immune deficiency syndrome: clinical findings, diagnosis and treatment, and review of the literature. *Medicine* (Baltimore) 1990;69:361-374.

13. Wheat LJ, Batteiger BE, Sathapatayavongs B: *Histoplasma capsulatum* infection of the central nervous system. *Medicine* 1990; 69:244-260.

14. Wheat LJ, Connolly-Stringfield P, Blair R, et al: Effect of successful treatment with amphotericin B on *Histoplasma capsulatum* variety *capsulatum* polysaccharide antigen levels in patients with AIDS and histoplasmosis. *Am J Med* 1992;92:153-160.

15. Wheat LJ, Hafner RE, Korzun AM, et al: Itraconazole treatment of disseminated histoplasmosis in patients with AIDS. *Am J Med* 1995;98:336-342.

16. Blanshard C, Ellis DS, Tovey DG, et al: Treatment of intestinal microsporidiosis with albendazole in patients with AIDS. *AIDS* 1992; 6:311-313.

17. Anwar-Bruni DM, Hogan SE, Schwartz DA, et al: Atovaquone is effective treatment for the symptoms of gastrointestinal microsporidiosis in HIV-1 infected patients. *AIDS* 1996;10:619-623.

18. Havlik JA, Horsburgh CR, Metchock B, et al: Disseminated *Mycobacterium avium* complex infection: clinical identification and epidemiologic trends. *J Infect Dis* 1992;165:577-580.

19. Jacobson MA, Hopewell PC, Yajko DM, et al: Natural history of disseminated *Mycobacterium avium* complex infection in AIDS. *J Infect Dis* 1991;164:994-998.

20. Chin DP, Hopewell PC, Yajko DM, et al: *Mycobacterium avium* complex in the respiratory or gastrointestinal tract and the risk of *M avium* complex bacteremia in patients with the human immunodeficiency virus. *J Infect Dis* 1994;169:289-295.

21. Chaisson RE, Benson CA, Dybe MP, et al: Clarithromycin therapy for bacteremic *Mycobacterium avium* complex disease: a randomized, double-blind, dose-ranging study in patients with AIDS. *Ann Intern Med* 1994;121:905-911.

22. Chaisson RE, Keiser P, Pierce M, et al: Clarithromycin and ethambutol with or without clofazimine for the treatment of bacteremic *Mycobacterium avium* complex disease in patients with HIV infection. *AIDS* 1997;11:311-317.

23. Snider DE Jr, Roper WL: The new tuberculosis. *N Engl J Med* 1992;326:703-705.

24. Hopewell PC: Tuberculosis in persons with human immunodeficiency virus infection. In: *The Medical Management of AIDS* Sande MA, Volberding PA, eds. Philadelphia, WB Saunders, 1997.

25. Onorato IM, McCray E, Field Services Branch: Prevalence of human immunodeficiency virus infection among patients attending tuberculosis clinics in the United States. *J Infect Dis* 1992;165:87-92.

26. Theuer CP, Hopewell PC, Elias D, et al: Human immunodeficiency virus infection in tuberculosis patients. *J Infect Dis* 1990;162:8-12.

27. American Thoracic Society: Control of tuberculosis in the United States. *Am Rev Resp Dis* 1992;146:1623-1633.

28. Jones BE, Young SM, Antoniskis D, et al: Relationship of the manifestations of tuberculosis to CD4 cell counts in patients with human immunodeficiency virus infection. *Am Rev Respir Dis* 1993;148:1292-1297.

29. Chin DP, Yajko DM, Hadley WK, et al: Clinical utility of a commercial test based on the polymerase chain reaction for detecting *Mycobacterium tuberculosis* in respiratory specimens. *Am J Respir Crit Care Med* 1995;151:1872-1877.

30. Iseman MD: Treatment of multidrug-resistant tuberculosis. *N Engl J Med* 1993;329:784-791.

31. Edman JC, Soglin ML: Molecular phylogeny of *Pneumocystis carinii*. In: Walzer PD, ed. *Pneumocystis carinii* Pneumonia. Vol 69. New York, Marcel Dekker Inc, 1994, pp 91-105.

32. Beard CB, Navin TR: Molecular epidemiology of *Pneumocystis carinii* pneumonia. *Emerg Infect Dis* 196;2:147-149.

33. Keely SP, Stringer JR, Baughman RP, et al: Genetic variation among *Pneumocystis carinii hominis* isolates in recurrent pneumocystosis. *J Infect Dis* 1995;172:595-598.

34. Phair J, Munoz A, Detels R, et al: The risk of *Pneumocystis carinii* pneumonia among men infected with human immunodeficiency virus type 1: the multicenter AIDS cohort study group. *N Engl J Med* 1990;322:161-165.

35. National Institutes of Health-University of California Expert Panel: Consensus statement on the use of corticosteroids as adjunctive therapy for severe *Pneumocystis carinii* pneumonia in the acquired immunodeficiency syndrome. *N Engl J Med* 1990;323:1500-1504.

36. Safrin S, Finkelstein DM, Feinberg J, et al: A double-blind, randomized comparison of oral trimethoprim-sulfamethoxazole, dapsone-trimethoprim, and clindamycin-primaquine for treatment of mild-to-moderate *Pneumocystis carinii* pneumonia in patients with AIDS. *Ann Intern Med* 1996;124:792-802.

37. Israelski DM, Chmiel JS, Poggensee L, et al: Prevalence of *Toxoplasma* infection in a cohort of homosexual men at risk of AIDS and toxoplasmic encephalitis. *J Acquir Immune Defic Syndr* 1993; 6:414-418.

38. Levy RM, Mills CM, Posin JP, et al: The efficacy and clinical impact of brain imaging in neurological symptomatic AIDS patients: a prospective CT/MRI study. *J Acquir Immune Defic Syndr* 1990;3:461-471.

39. Canessa A, Del Bono V, De Leo P, et al: Cotrimoxazole therapy of *Toxoplasma gondii* encephalitis in AIDS patients. *Eur J Clin Microbiol Infect Dis* 1992;11:125-130.

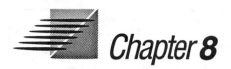

Chapter 8

Treatment of Cytomegalovirus Disease

Cytomegalovirus (CMV) disease remains a significant problem for patients with advanced AIDS. Before the advent of highly active antiretroviral therapies with combinations of drugs that include protease inhibitors and nucleoside analog reverse transcriptase inhibitors, approximately 40% of patients with CD4+ cell counts below 50/mm³ were likely to develop cytomegalovirus disease: primarily retinitis, and to a lesser extent, gastrointestinal and pulmonary disease.[1] While the incidence of CMV disease may be decreasing, it remains a significant problem for those patients who have failed the highly active regimens, and even for some of those who had an initial CD4+ cell count response.[2] The treatment options for cytomegalovirus disease recently expanded to include one new drug and several novel delivery systems. The development of oral prodrugs that have significantly better bioavailability is well underway, although none is available yet.

Three drugs have been approved to treat cytomegalovirus retinitis: cidofovir (Vistide®), foscarnet (Foscavir®), and ganciclovir (Cytovene®) (Figure 1). Although all of these treatments were originally developed and can be prescribed as intravenous formulations, ganciclovir is also available in oral and intravitreal formulations, and is the active agent in

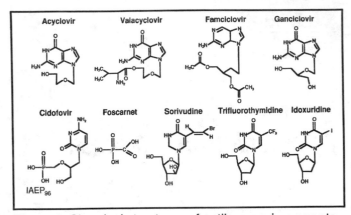

Figure 1: Chemical structures of antiherpesvirus agents. Ganciclovir, foscarnet, and cidofovir have clinically relevant anticytomegalovirus activity.

an approved intravitreal sustained-release device (Vitrasert®). An oral prodrug is in clinical development. Foscarnet is available as an intravitreal treatment; development of an oral formulation has been unsuccessful. Cidofovir is recommended to be administered intravenously only. Initial reports of success with intravitreal cidofovir have been tempered by recent data suggesting that this approach may be too toxic.

Therapeutic Options for Patients Newly Diagnosed With Cytomegalovirus Retinitis

Initiating therapy in a patient newly diagnosed with CMV retinitis can be successfully accomplished by a variety of treatment approaches. Although each approach is predictably associated with different toxicities and management concerns, all are effective. The decision to use one therapy or another has become individualized and depends on the patient's understanding of expected benefits and risks, and the attending physician's familiarity with the specific treatment. In general, treatment is more intense during the first 2 weeks of therapy (induction therapy). After the retinitis stabilizes, usually within 14 to 21 days, a chronic maintenance therapy is administered indefinitely at a reduced dosage. The following CMV therapies have been shown to be effective in patients with newly diagnosed and relapsed retinitis.

Cidofovir

Cidofovir is a nucleotide analog that is active against all of the herpesviruses, including drug-resistant CMV. As a nucleotide, it appears to the infected cell as a monophosphate that does not require the viral enzyme necessary for the first monophosphorylation step. This is important because it can be used against ganciclovir-resistant mutations. However, it is also capable of producing toxicity in uninfected cells.

Another important property of cidofovir is its prolonged intracellular half-life. Cidofovir induction is only required weekly, and maintenance therapy is needed biweekly. Unfortunately, cidofovir is nephrotoxic, and may cause renal tubular acidosis or Fanconi's syndrome. Probenecid (Benemid®) must be administered before and after cidofovir infusion to block the absorption of the drug into the proximal tubule, thus providing a measure of protection against renal damage. Vigorous hydration is critical.

Three studies have been completed that demonstrate the clinical efficacy of cidofovir. The Studies of the Ocular Complications of AIDS (SOCA) group treated 64 patients with newly diagnosed peripheral retinitis. Patients were treated with a high dose of cidofovir, 5 mg/kg, a lower dose, 3 mg/kg, or had their treatment deferred. Treatment was weekly for 2 weeks, then every 2 weeks thereafter. The deferral group experienced expected progression of their retinitis in the 21 days, the low-dose group progressed in a median of 69 days, and the high-dose group never reached a median progression before the study was completed. The rates of visual loss were similar between treatment groups. Two patients in the high-dose group experienced partially reversible renal insufficiency. Probenecid reactions were common.[3]

Study 106 compared the cidofovir 5-mg/kg dosing regimen with treatment deferral in patients with newly diagnosed peripheral retinitis. In this study, patients who received treatment experienced retinitis progression in 120 days, compared with only 22 days for those who deferred therapy. Proteinuria was common (15%) in the treated patients. Other side effects included neutropenia (15%), increased creatinine (7%), nausea/vomiting (38%), fever/chills (28%), rash (18%), headache (13%), asthenia (13%), and myalgia (8%).[4]

A third trial was designed as a salvage study for patients who had failed ganciclovir or foscarnet therapy. Sixty patients were assigned to receive 3- or 5-mg/kg dosing regimens of cidofovir, weekly for the first 2 weeks, then every 2 weeks. The time to progression of retinitis in the 5-mg group was 115 days, compared with 49 days for the 3-mg treatment group. As observed in other trials, therapy was associated with proteinuria and increases in serum creatinine.[5]

Cidofovir is effective and safe in newly diagnosed and previously treated patients when they are monitored closely for proteinuria and renal insufficiency. The obvious advantage of cidofovir is that it requires only infrequent dosing and, therefore, does not necessitate an indwelling central vein catheter. A disadvantage, however, is that renal toxicity and probenecid reactions are common, but can be successfully managed in most instances.

Cidofovir Administration

Induction therapy: 5 mg/kg/wk for 2 consecutive weeks intravenously at a constant rate over 1 hour. To prevent significant renal toxicity, probenecid must be administered orally before every dose. Two grams must be given 3 hours before the first dose, and 1 gram given 2 hours and again at 8 hours after cidofovir administration. Because probenecid often is poorly tolerated, we advise that all administrations of probenecid be observed by a trained health-care worker.

Maintenance therapy: 5 mg/kg every 2 weeks indefinitely, administered as above with probenecid.

Pros: Cidofovir is an effective therapy.[3-5] Intravenous administration weekly and then every other week can be done without a semipermanent intravenous access device. By avoiding a central venous line, patients are spared inconvenience, expense, and risk of infection. Although many clinicians rightfully insist on administering cidofovir in the outpatient setting (ie, not in the home), the overall frequency is not terribly cumbersome, approximately twice a month.

Cons: Cidofovir and probenecid can be highly toxic. Dose-dependent nephrotoxicity to cidofovir is the most significant dose-limiting toxicity. In some patients, renal function did not return to normal after drug discontinuation. Cidofovir should be discontinued if proteinuria or decreased renal function is observed. Cidofovir should not be initiated in patients with serum creatinine >1.5 mg/dL or creatinine clearance $\leq$ 55 mL/min. Cidofovir-associated neutropenia and metabolic acidosis also have been reported. Probenecid reactions occur in approximately half of patients and include rash, nausea, vomiting, and fever. It is critical that all doses of probenecid be administered as recommended and that patients are well hydrated on the day of cidofovir administration.

Foscarnet

Foscarnet (phosphonoformic acid) is structurally very different from all of the drugs used to treat herpesvirus infections (Figure 1). Foscarnet is not metabolized and is excreted unchanged in the urine. Foscarnet directly inhibits CMV DNA polymerase and does not require phosphorylation by viral or cellular enzymes.

In a comparison with ganciclovir therapy in patients with newly diagnosed retinitis, the time to disease progression was similar, although survival was better (12.6 compared with 8.5 months; P=0.006) in patients assigned foscarnet (Figure 2).[6] Foscarnet has not been compared to cidofovir in a controlled study.

The primary side effect of foscarnet is renal insufficiency. This well-known problem usually can be avoided by careful hydration. Electrolytes, which are often altered during treat-

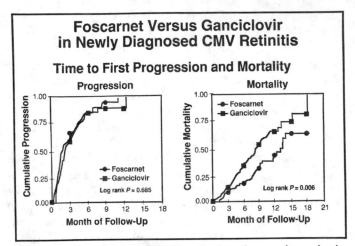

Figure 2: The time to retinitis progression and survival in patients newly diagnosed with cytomegalovirus retinitis treated with foscarnet or ganciclovir.[6]

ment, can be replaced, typically with oral supplements.[7] The inhibition of foscarnet is dose dependent, as is the survival benefit observed in some clinical studies.[8] As a result, many clinicians routinely use the maximum recommended dose of foscarnet, 120 mg/kg/d. Although resistance to foscarnet occurs, CMV more readily develops resistance to ganciclovir.

Foscarnet Administration

Induction therapy: 90-120 mg/kg every 12 hours for 14 to 21 days (dose adjusted for renal function). Administration should be by infusion pump over a minimum of 1 hour. Tolerance of the infusion may be enhanced if the drug is administered over a longer period, such as 2 hours. The patient should be adequately hydrated.

Maintenance therapy: 90-120 mg/kg/d, infused as above. A survival advantage has been observed with the 120 mg/kg dosage.[8]

Pros: Foscarnet is an effective therapy and has been associated in one study with improved survival compared with therapy with intravenous ganciclovir.[6] In addition to having an effect on CMV, foscarnet also has activity against other herpesviruses, including acyclovir-resistant herpes simplex. There is also a modest effect against HIV-1 and hepatitis B. Less resistance to foscarnet has been observed compared with ganciclovir.

Cons: The most significant toxicity of foscarnet is renal impairment, defined as a rise in serum creatinine to 2 mg/dL or greater, which occurs in up to 33% of patients. Renal impairment is usually reversible after discontinuation of foscarnet. Electrolyte imbalances may be observed in up to 15% of patients and may require oral or parenteral supplementation. Seizures have been reported in patients receiving foscarnet; however, most were attributable to other causes related to HIV-1 infection and not to foscarnet.[7] A chronic indwelling venous catheter is required for the daily maintenance infusions.

Ganciclovir

The first anti-CMV therapy was ganciclovir, a nucleoside analog very similar in structure to acyclovir (Zovirax®). As with all nucleoside analogs, ganciclovir must be triphosphorylated before its incorporation as a substrate for viral DNA polymerase. Triphosphorylation occurs stepwise when the first monophosphorylation step is catalyzed by a CMV enzyme with active protein kinase, which is a product of the CMV UL97 gene. The subsequent steps are processed by cellular enzymes. Resistance to ganciclovir most commonly arises from mutations in the viral enzyme rather than in the viral DNA polymerase.

Ganciclovir can cause profound bone marrow suppression. However, granulocytopenia and anemia generally can be successfully treated with cytokines such as filgastrim (recombinant human granulocyte colony stimulating factor G-CSF, Neupogen®) or epoetin alfa (Procrit®, Epogen®).

Therapy with intravenous ganciclovir has been compared to intravenous foscarnet (Figure 2), the time to retinitis progression being equivalent. An oral formulation of ganciclovir has been approved as maintenance therapy, although results are inferior to those observed with intravenous delivery.[9,10] Oral ganciclovir is also approved as a prophylactic agent in patients at high risk for CMV disease (CD4+ cell count <50/mm³). However, neutropenia, anemia, limited efficacy, lack of improvement in survival, and cost are among the issues that should be considered in decisions to initiate this form of prophylaxis.[11,12]

An implantable intraocular device (Vitrasert®) that contains ganciclovir with a continuous release of drug for 6 or more months has recently been approved. Treatment with this implant has resulted in much higher intravitreal drug concentrations compared with systemic administration. Efficacy is better with implants than with other therapies. In two randomized trials, the median times to progression were virtually equal to the period of drug release.[13,14] Complications of the implantable intraocular device include a transient decrease in visual acuity, retinal detachment, intravitreal hemorrhage, and endophthalmitis. Because the implant is only a local therapy, systemic treatment for prevention of infection in the contralateral eye and other body organs is recommended.

Ganciclovir Administration

Induction therapy: 5 mg/kg every 12 hours intravenously over 1 hour for 14 to 21 days is an effective therapy (dose adjusted for renal insufficiency). The oral formulation should not be used for induction therapy.

Maintenance therapy: 5 mg/kg/d, should continue indefinitely. Alternatively, oral ganciclovir, 1000 mg t.i.d. can be used, although efficacy is better with the intravenous administration because oral ganciclovir is poorly absorbed.

Maintenance therapy with Vitrasert®: 4.5 mg of ganciclovir is released at a constant rate of 1 µg/h. The device is inserted surgically by making a small incision in the avascular pars plana area of the sclera under local anesthesia. The device is held in place by a single suture. The device must be replaced approximately every 6 months.

Pros: Ganciclovir is an effective therapy. Oral ganciclovir, although not quite as effective as the intravenous formulation, does avoid the necessity of an indwelling central venous catheter, as does the ganciclovir intravitreal insert. The infusions are generally well tolerated and do not require an infusion pump. The intravitreal device is associated with longest disease-free survival in the affected eye.[13,14]

Cons: Ganciclovir is associated with neutropenia, anemia, and thrombocytopenia, often requiring the use of cytokines such as filgastrim to raise the neutrophil count to safe levels. The ganciclovir intraocular device alone places patients at high risk for the development of contralateral retinitis and visceral disease and, therefore, should be used in conjunction with some form of systemic therapy. Visual acuity is temporarily lowered after surgical insertion of the intraocular device, which must be done in a surgical setting. Retinal detachment has a higher incidence in the early postoperative period. Oral ganciclovir is poorly absorbed and should not be used in sight-threatening disease or if malabsorption is expected. Viral resistance, although uncommon, is more likely with ganciclovir than with foscarnet. The intravenous formulation necessitates the placement of a chronic indwelling catheter.

Therapeutic Options of Patients With Relapsing CMV Disease

Although all of the therapies listed above can be used for the treatment of relapsing CMV disease, additional therapeutic approaches include combinations of anti-CMV drugs. The only combination studied is ganciclovir plus foscarnet. The systemic administration has been investigated the most thoroughly.

Combination Therapy With Ganciclovir Plus Foscarnet

Because of improved antiretroviral therapy and treatment of other HIV-1 related complications, AIDS patients are living longer, including those with active CMV disease. Some patients have experienced six or more relapses of CMV retinitis or have developed CMV disease elsewhere, which indicates a need for even better therapies.

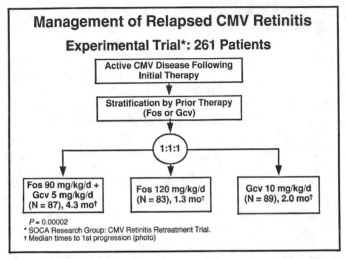

Figure 3: Study design and time to relapse of retinitis in patients who experienced at least one prior relapse, and then treated with either foscarnet 120 mg/kg/d, ganciclovir 10 mg/kg/d, or the combination foscarnet 90 mg/kg/d plus ganciclovir 5 mg/kg/d. The Cytomegalovirus Retreatment Trial, SOCA.[17]

One potential therapeutic option is treatment with both ganciclovir and foscarnet, a combination that is synergistic in vitro. When administered to patients who were unresponsive to either drug given alone, a better treatment response than expected was observed.[15,16] The combination of systemic ganciclovir and foscarnet has been examined in a prospective study, the CMV Retinitis Retreatment Trial (CRRT). The CRRT enrolled 279 eligible patients with AIDS and relapsing CMV retinitis. The average number of prior relapses was slightly less than two. Patients were randomized to receive maintenance doses of either foscarnet 120 mg/kg, ganciclovir 10 mg/kg, or the combination foscarnet 90 mg/kg and ganciclovir 5 mg/kg daily. Although ganciclovir and foscarnet can not be infused simultaneously, they can be administered sequentially or at different times.

The principal results of the CRRT are presented in Figure 3. In the results from the masked fundus reading center, the time to first CMV relapse was 1.3, 2.0, and 4.3 months for the foscarnet, ganciclovir and combination groups respectively (P=0.001). Survival was similar for all groups, ranging from 8.4 to 9.0 months.

The CRRT protocol evaluated several ocular measures. There was a difference in the monthly rate of change in the involved retinal area in favor of the combination group, 1.19% compared with 1.4% and 2.47% for the ganciclovir and foscarnet monotherapy groups (P=0.04). Visual field and the rate in change of visual field also favored the combination treatment. There was no difference in visual acuity. Interestingly, the occurrence of adverse events was similar in the three treatment groups.[17]

Intraocular Injection

Limited experience has been reported with intraocular injections of ganciclovir or foscarnet in combination with systemic administration of other anti-CMV agents. The most commonly used drug for intraocular injection is ganciclovir. Doses of 400 to 2000 µg in a volume of 0.1 mm^3 have been successfully administered from 1 to 3 times per week. Foscarnet also has been given by intraocular injection. Doses of 2400 µg have been administered safely, but may have to be given more frequently than ganciclovir injections.[18,19] Intraocular injection for CMV retinitis has the advantage of providing high concentrations of drug to the infected site. Disadvantages include infection and discomfort with the procedure, which must be repeated 1 to 3 times per week.

Conclusion

Systemic and local anti-CMV therapy with ganciclovir, foscarnet, and cidofovir are now options for patients with many forms of CMV disease. As patients' overall prognoses continue to improve, clinicians will be forced to use various treatments to control CMV disease. A firm understanding of the benefits and risks of these therapies is essential for clinicians managing patients with CMV disease.

References

1. Hoover DR, Saah AJ, Bacellar H, et al: Clinical manifestations of AIDS in the era of *Pneumocystis* prophylaxis. *N Engl J Med* 1993;329:1922-1926.

2. Jacobson MA, Kramer R, Pavan PR, et al: Failure of highly active antiretroviral therapy (HAART) to prevent CMV retinitis despite marked CD4 count increases. In: Abstracts of the 4th Conference on Retroviruses and Opportunistic Infections. Washington, DC, January 22-26, 1997. [abstract 353]

3. Studies of Ocular Complications of AIDS Research Group in collaboration with the AIDS Clinical Trials Group: Parenteral cidofovir for cytomegalovirus retinitis in patients with AIDS: the HPMPC peripheral cytomegalovirus retinitis trial. A randomized, controlled trial. *Ann Intern Med* 1997;126:264-274.

4. Lalezari JP, Stagg RJ, Kuppermann BD, et al: Intravenous cidofovir for peripheral cytomegalovirus retinitis in patients with AIDS. A randomized, controlled trial. *Ann Intern Med* 1997;126:257-263.

5. Lalezari JP, Kemper C, Stagg R, et al: A randomized, controlled study of the safety and efficacy of intravenous cidofovir (CDV, HPMPC) for the treatment of relapsing cytomegalovirus retinitis in patients with AIDS. In: Abstracts of the 11th International Conference on AIDS. Vancouver, July 7-12, 1997. [Abstract Th.B.304]

6. Studies of Ocular Complications of AIDS Research Group in collaboration with the AIDS Clinical Trials Group: Mortality in patients with the acquired immunodeficiency syndrome treated with either foscarnet or ganciclovir for cytomegalovirus retinitis. *N Engl J Med* 1992;326:213-220.

7. Studies of Ocular Complications of AIDS Research Group in collaboration with the AIDS Clinical Trials Group: Morbidity and toxic effects associated with ganciclovir or foscarnet therapy in a randomized cytomegalovirus retinitis trial. *Arch Intern Med* 1995;155:65-74.

8. Jacobson MA, Causey D, Polsky B, et al: A dose-ranging study of daily maintenance intravenous foscarnet therapy for cytomegalovirus retinitis in AIDS. *J Infect Dis* 1993;168:444-448.

9. Drew WL, Ives D, Lalezari JP, et al: Oral ganciclovir as maintenance treatment for cytomegalovirus retinitis in patients with AIDS. *N Engl J Med* 1995;333:615-620.

10. The Oral Ganciclovir European and Australian Cooperative Study Group: Intravenous versus oral ganciclovir: European/Australian comparative study of efficacy and safety in the prevention of cytomegalovirus retinitis recurrence in patients with AIDS. *AIDS* 1995;9:471-477.

11. Spector SA, McKinley GF, Lalezari JP, et al: Oral ganciclovir for the prevention of cytomegalovirus disease in persons with AIDS. *N Engl J Med* 1996;334:1491-1497.

12. Centers for Disease Control and Prevention: 1997 USPHS/IDSA guidelines for the prevention of opportunistic infections in persons infected with human immunodeficiency virus. *MMWR* 1997;46:1-46.

13. Martin DF, Parks DJ, Mellow SD, et al: Treatment of cytomegalovirus retinitis with an intraocular sustained-release ganciclovir implant. *Arch Ophthalmol* 1994;112:1531-1539.

14. Musch DC, Martin DF, Gordon JF, et al: Treatment of cytomegalovirus retinitis with a sustained-release ganciclovir implant. The Ganciclovir Implant Study Group. *N Engl J Med* 1997;337:83-90.

15. Dieterich DT, Poles MA, Lew EA, et al: Concurrent use of ganciclovir and foscarnet to treat cytomegalovirus infection in AIDS patients. *J Infect Dis* 1993;167:1184-1188.

16. Weinberg DV, Murphy R, Naughton K: Combined daily therapy with intravenous ganciclovir and foscarnet for patients with recurrent cytomegalovirus retinitis. *Am J Ophthalmol* 1994;117:776-782.

17. The Studies of Ocular Complications of AIDS Research Group in collaboration with the AIDS Clinical Trials Group: Combination foscarnet and ganciclovir therapy vs monotherapy for the treatment of relapsed cytomegalovirus retinitis in patients with AIDS. The Cytomegalovirus Retreatment Trial. *Arch Ophthalmol* 1996;114:23-33.

18. Masur H, Whitcup SM, Cartwright C, et al: Advances in the management of AIDS-related cytomegalovirus retinitis. *Ann Intern Med* 1996;125:126-136.

19. Jacobson MA: Treatment of cytomegalovirus retinitis in patients with the acquired immunodeficiency syndrome. *N Engl J Med* 1997;337:105-114.

Chapter 9

Wasting in HIV Infection

Weight loss, or wasting, is an important complication of HIV-1 infection. In fact, in Africa, AIDS has been termed the "slim disease." The causes of wasting in patients with HIV-1 have been extensively investigated. Weight loss can be caused by: (1) gastrointestinal infection with opportunistic pathogens that leads to diarrhea and malabsorption; (2) opportunistic infections such as *Pneumocystis carinii* pneumonia (PCP); (3) endocrine and metabolic alterations; and (4) depression resulting in loss of appetite and decreased calorie intake. Studies of starvation have firmly documented that malnutrition impairs immune function. In persons infected with HIV-1, wasting impairs performance, quality of life, and survival.[1-3] In a retrospective analysis, the risk of death was increased 8-fold in men who had lost 10% of body weight and, in the Multicenter AIDS Cohort Study (MACS), weight loss of greater than 10% before the diagnosis of AIDS reduced survival significantly after the onset of an AIDS-defining event.[2,3] Tables 1 and 2 outline causes and treatment of AIDS-related weight loss.

Many HIV-1 infected individuals become infected with enteric pathogens or develop malignant disease that can result in anorexia, dysphagia, odynophagia, diarrhea, malabsorption, and, ultimately, malnutrition. Common infections

Table 1: Causes of Weight Loss in AIDS

- Anorexia
- Uncontrolled opportunistic infection
- Malabsorption
- Altered metabolism

Table 2: Treatment of Wasting Syndrome

- Treat infection
- Stimulate appetite
- Anabolic steroids plus exercise
- Treat hypogonadism, if present

of the upper gastrointestinal tract include oropharyngeal candidiasis, esophagitis from candidiasis, cytomegalovirus (CMV), and herpes simplex. Symptoms include anorexia from taste alteration, dysphagia, odynophagia, or esophageal spasm. Diagnosis of the cause of esophageal infections requires endoscopy, biopsy, and culture. Treatment of esophagitis from candidiasis with antifungal agents is usually associated with a good response unless the infection is caused by *Candida* species that are resistant to the imidazoles, in which case therapy with intravenous amphotericin B (Fungizone®) is necessary. Treatment with the antiviral agents ganciclovir (Cytovene®), foscarnet (Foscavir®), and acyclovir (Zovirax®) also usually controls symptoms of viral esophagitis.[4]

Although the cause of aphthous ulcers of the oropharynx is not known, studies have demonstrated that these painful lesions, which can inhibit oral intake, respond to thalidomide. Aphthous ulceration of the esophagus can also reduce calorie intake because of odynophagia. The response of the aphthous ulcers in this location to thalidomide has not been clearly defined. In addition to hemorrhage, non-Hodgkin's lymphoma of the stomach can be associated with outlet obstruction and can interfere with eating. Although Kaposi's sarcoma of the stomach is common and occasionally causes hemorrhage, it does not often cause gastrointestinal symptoms. The hepatobiliary system can be infected by the agents commonly complicating advanced HIV-1 infection. *Cryptosporidium* can produce cholecystitis. Cytomegalovirus is a well-recognized cause of hepatitis and can produce cholecystitis and obstruction of the common duct.[4]

Diarrhea is the major cause of gastrointestinal disease that leads to wasting. The range of causes is extensive and includes CMV, *Mycobacterium avium* complex, *Cryptosporidium*, *Entamoeba histolytica*, *Giardia lamblia*, *Isospora bella*, *Salmonella*, *Clostridium difficile*, *Campylobacter*, and other enteric pathogens. The evaluation of patients with diarrhea requires culture for bacteria pathogens, a search for ova and parasites, and, often, endoscopic studies with biopsy. Thorough investigation, however, might not identify a cause of the diarrhea. HIV-1 infection of enterocytes leading to villous atrophy and malabsorption of fat or D-xylose is thought to be the cause.[4]

As in all patients with severe infections, HIV-1 infected individuals lose weight, particularly because of the complicating opportunistic infections. Patients will often lose 5% of their ideal weight during an episode of PCP and regain this weight, incompletely, after clearing of the pneumonia. Acute infection in HIV-1 infected patients is not associated with a reduction in resting energy expenditure, a compensatory mechanism that slows weight loss during acute infections in patients not infected with HIV-1.[5] Asymptomatic HIV-1 infected persons also have been shown to have reduced both calorie intake and total energy expenditure,[6] both of which contribute to loss of lean body mass. In addition, endocrinopathies have been described that contribute to loss of muscle, especially in persons with advanced HIV-1 infection. Hypogonadism has been well documented in men with advanced HIV-1 disease, but other hormonal deficiencies are uncommon, especially in asymptomatic individuals.[7,8] Other conditions that should be identified in patients losing weight are adrenal insufficiency from CMV adrenalitis, ketoconazole-induced impairment of steroidogenesis, and rifampin-induced increased cortisol catabolism. Diabetes, as a consequence of didanosine (ddI)- or pentamidine-induced pancreatitis, also is not uncommon.

The role of cytokine dysregulation in HIV-1 induced wasting has not been defined completely. Tumor necrosis factor-alpha (TNF) secretion and interleukin-1 are upregulated and both are thought to contribute to protein catabolism.[8] Attempts to reduce TNF production with thalidomide or other pharmacologic agents such as pentoxyfylline (Trental®) have not been effective in preventing wasting.

The management of patients with HIV-1 infection and wasting should first focus on ruling out treatable causes of diarrhea, then on searching for and treating chronic complicating infections or neoplasms such as disseminated MAC infection or non-Hodgkin's lymphoma, and finally, on identifying possible endocrine deficiencies. If no complication can be identified, the patient may benefit from the use of appetite stimulants, anabolic steroids, or exercise. Patients' appetites can be increased by the administration of megestrol acetate (Megace®) or dronabinol (Marinol®).[9,10] Unfortunately, the weight gain produced by these stimulants is predominantly fat rather than lean body mass. Furthermore, megestrol therapy has been associated with testosterone deficiency.[11] Also, it has been observed that transient adrenal insufficiency occurs after discontinuation of this progestational agent.[8]

An increase in lean body mass has long been noted with administration of anabolic steroids, both in HIV-1 infected patients and noninfected individuals. More recently, recombinant human growth hormone (rHgh) was demonstrated to increase lean body mass as opposed to just increasing body weight. This benefit was associated with augmented endurance and an improved sense of well-being. Concomitant increases in retention of nitrogen with administration of these anabolic steroids or rHgh has been documented as well.[12]

Trials are underway to evaluate combining appetite stimulants with anabolic agents to determine if retention of lean body mass can be optimized in HIV-1 infected patients who have just begun to lose weight. Clinicians must recognize that although weight loss is a risk factor for disease progression and that profound wasting is associated with increased mortality, research has not definitively documented that reversing weight loss improves immune function or slows progression of HIV-1 infection in the absence of effective antiretroviral therapy.

References

1. Beisel WR: Malnutrition as a consequence of stress. In: Suskind RM, ed. *Malnutrition and the Immune Response*. Chapter 3. New York, Raven Press, 1997.

2. Guenther P, Muurahainen U, Kosok A, et al: Relationships among nutritional states, disease progression and survival in HIV infection. *J Acquir Immune Defic Syndr* 1993;6:1130-1138.

3. Palenicek JG, Graham NM, He YD, et al: Weight loss prior to clinical AIDS as a predictor of survival. *J AIDS Hum Retrovir* 1995;10:336-373.

4. Cello JP: Gastrointestinal tract manifestations of AIDS. In: Sande MA, Volberding P, eds. *The Medical Management of AIDS*. 4th ed. Philadelphia, WB Saunders Co, 1995, pp 241-260.

5. Grunfeld C, Pang M, Shime L, et al: Resting energy expenditure, calorie intake and short-term weight change in human immunodeficiency syndrome. *Am J Clin Nutr* 1992;55:455-460.

6. Macallan DC, Noble C, Baldwin C, et al: Energy expenditure and wasting in human immunodeficiency virus infection. *N Engl J Med* 1995;333:83-88.

7. Dobs AS, Dempsey MA, Lodenson PW, et al: Endocrine disorders in men infected with human immunodeficiency virus. *Am J Med* 1988;84:611-616.

8. Grenspoon SK, Donovoan DS, Bilezikian JP: Aetiology and pathogenesis of hormonal and metabolic disorders in HIV infection. In: Norbialo G, ed. *The Endocrinology and Metabolism of HIV Infection*. Baillierés, Clinical Endocrinology and Metabolism, 1994;4:735-756.

9. Goster R, Seefried M, Volberding P: Dronabinol effects on weight in patients with HIV infection. *AIDS* 1992;6;127.

10. Von Roenn JH, Amstrong DA, Kotler DP, et al: Megestrol acetate in patients with AIDS-related cachexia. *Ann Intern Med* 1994; 121:393-399.

11. Engelson ES, Tierney AR, PI-Sunyer FX, et al: Effects of megestrol acetate upon body composition and circulating testosterone in patients with AIDS. *J AIDS Hum Retrovir* 1995;9:1107-7108.

12. Mulligan K, Grunfeld C, Hellenstein MK, et al: Anabolic effects of recombinant human growth hormone in patients with wasting associated with human immunodeficiency infection. *J Clin Endocrinol Metab* 1993;77:956-962.

Chapter 10

Central Nervous System Manifestations of HIV Infection

HIV-1 commonly affects the neurologic system, as do opportunistic infections and neoplastic complications of the immunosuppression induced by the retrovirus. Many of these conditions are relatively uncommon in people without HIV-1 infection, most of whom respond poorly to specific treatment even if proven therapy is available.[1] Table 1 outlines some of these conditions.

During primary HIV-1 infection, a small number of patients have signs and symptoms of viral meningitis. Examination of the cerebrospinal fluid (CSF) reveals pleocytosis and elevated protein seen in the typical patient with aseptic meningitis.[2] The illness is generally self-limited and, with recovery, patients enter the clinically latent period of HIV-1 infection. Less commonly, patients may have encephalitis or cranial neuropathies. An ascending polyneuropathy similar to Guillain-Barré syndrome is also seen in patients with acute HIV-1 infection.

Examination of the CSF of patients in the clinically latent phase of HIV-1 infection sometimes demonstrates modest mononuclear cell pleocytosis and elevations of protein, which suggest that the virus infects the central nervous system (CNS) early in the course of most HIV-1 cases.[3] These findings also suggest that HIV-1 is not directly cytopathic for

Table 1: Central Nervous System Manifestations of HIV-1 Infection

Acute HIV-1 infection:
- viral meningitis
- encephalitis
- ascending polyneuropathy

Opportunistic infections (late HIV-1 infection):
- *Toxoplasma* cerebritis
- cryptococcal meningitis
- progressive multifocal leukoencephalopathy
- neurosyphilis
- *Mycobacterium tuberculosis* meningitis
- cytomegalovirus encephalitis
- herpes simplex encephalitis

Neoplastic disease (late HIV-1 infection):
- CNS lymphoma
- Kaposi's sarcoma

AIDS dementia complex

neurons and that the ascending neuropathies may be caused by autoimmune mechanisms. One of the most common neurologic complications, reactivation of herpes zoster infection (shingles), often heralds the termination of the clinically latent phase of HIV-1 infection. The onset of shingles can be seen in patients with $CD4^+$ lymphocyte counts of 400 to 500/mm^3. Mononeuritis multiplex is much less common and, if it occurs early in HIV-1 infection, usually has a benign course. A late occurrence can be more severe and can lead to paralysis.

Most neurologic complications of HIV-1 infection occur in patients with advanced immunosuppression.[4] The opportunistic infections include cryptococcal meningitis, tuberculosis meningitis, neurosyphilis, *Toxoplasma* cerebritis, progressive multifocal leukoencephalopathy, viral encephalitis caused by cytomegalovirus (CMV), herpes simplex, and, less commonly, herpes zoster. The management of cryptococcal meningitis and toxoplasmosis is described in Chapter 7, which outlines treatment of opportunistic infections.

Progressive multifocal leukoencephalopathy (PML) caused by the JC polyoma virus was rarely diagnosed before the HIV-1 epidemic and was usually seen in patients with suppression of cell-mediated immunity from Hodgkin's lymphoma. It presents with cognitive disturbances, such as a difficulty finding the right word. Imaging scans locate the usually multifocal lesions of PML in the white matter and they progress over a matter of weeks. Clinical progression parallels increasing involvement of the CNS as documented by imaging techniques, and most patients succumb in 1 to 3 months after diagnosis. The cells infected with the JC papova virus are the oligodendrocytes and the pathology is characterized by demyelination.[5,6] Although treatment with cytosine arabinoside (Cytosar-U, Tarabine PF5) has been suggested to stabilize PML,[7] the AIDS Clinical Trials Group (ACTG) study failed to demonstrate a benefit with either systemic or local therapy administered intraventricularly via an Ommaya reservoir.

Encephalitis caused by CMV is increasingly recognized as a late CNS infection. Although CNS CMV infection is probably common, only the occasional patient will manifest a clinical picture consistent with encephalitis. Cytomegalovirus myelitis with neurologic defects related to the spinal cord lesions is also increasingly recognized by clinicians caring for patients with advanced HIV-1 infection.[8] In these patients, aggressive treatment with the combination of ganciclovir (Cytovene®) and foscarnet (Foscavir®) may stabilize the neurologic status, but the long-term prognosis is very poor. Similarly, although herpetic encephalitis has been documented to occur with HIV-1 infection, the frequency and importance of this complication remain to be defined. Treatment with acyclovir (Zovirax®) is indicated in cases with disease confirmed by biopsy. Diagnosis of both of these complicating viral infections in the CNS may be greatly facilitated with the polymerase chain reaction (PCR) to detect the specific viral DNA in cerebrospinal fluid.[9]

The management of CNS lymphoma is described in Chapter 11 on neoplastic complications of HIV-1. Other less common focal neurologic complications include cryptococcoma, tuberculous brain abscess, and vascular disorders. The pathogenesis of the transient ischemic attacks or completed strokes is not clear, but thrombotic emboli are implicated in some patients.[10] The use of imaging techniques has greatly increased the ability to diagnose focal disorders and to manage patients with them. Except for vascular disease, most focal disorders, CNS lymphoma, toxoplasmosis, and PML evolve subacutely over several weeks. The characteristics and location of the lesion detected with an MRI often strongly suggest the diagnosis and lead to an immediate biopsy or therapeutic trial, as with suspected toxoplasmosis.

The most common diffuse encephalopathy in patients with HIV-1 infection is the AIDS Dementia Complex (ADC) manifested by cognitive, motor, and behavioral alterations.[11] Usually, the encephalopathy is seen in patients with a diagnosis of AIDS, although approximately 7% present with ADC. The dementia is characterized by mental status changes and slowing of motor function, both of which can be detected with formal neuropsychologic studies. Although a single evaluation may not detect loss of function for those with a high degree of education, serial studies show progressive subclinical declines. Loss of function is more easily detected in less educated individuals who appear to be less able to compensate for minor deficits of cognitive function.[12] The patient with ADC usually will first lose the ability to concentrate; often, the first symptom is difficulty with balancing a checkbook. Memory is also affected; appointments are missed and the patient reports the need to keep lists as a reminder. Although responses to questions may be slowed, the results of the bedside mental status examination can remain normal until there has been more marked progression. Motor skills may become impaired, especially of the hands, as the dementia progresses. Reports of dropping small objects are common and rapid hand motions are slowed, as can be detected on examination. Some patients develop ataxia at a later stage, but incontinence usually is not seen until just before the patient enters a vegetative status. The pathology associated with the ADC is focused in the subcortical structures and marked by gliosis, astrocytosis, and multinucleated giant cells. Histologic signs of inflammation are notably absent. In the spinal cord, vascular myelopathy is a prominent finding with or without the giant cells formed from infected macrophages and microglia cells.[13]

Imaging studies are required to rule out other causes of CNS dysfunction and usually demonstrate cerebral atrophy. Cerebrospinal fluid findings include the pleocytosis and elevated protein found in most patients with HIV-1 infection. β_2-microglobulin and neopterin, markers of immune activation, are elevated in CSF in patients with dementia from HIV-1.[14] There are reports of stabilization and even improvement in cognitive function in some patients who receive zidovudine, but the prevalence of ADC apparently has not decreased with the more widespread use of effective antiretroviral therapy.[4] The major investigative requirements are the need to determine the ability of newer agents to cross the blood-brain barrier and to more rigorously document the effect of highly effective antiretroviral compounds to prevent the dementia from developing or to reverse the neurologic changes after they commence.

References

1. McArthur JC: Neurologic diseases associated with HIV-1 infection. *Curr Opin Inf Dis* 1995;8:74-84.

2. Cooper DA, Gold J, McLean P, et al: Acute AIDS retrovirus infection; definition of a clinical illness associated with seroconversion. *Lancet* 1985;1:537-540.

3. Hollander H, Stringari S: Human immunodeficiency virus-associated meningitis: clinical course and correlations. *Am J Med* 1987; 83:813-816.

4. Bacellar H, Muñoz A, Miller EN, et al: Temporal trends in the incidence of HIV-1 related neurologic disease: MACS 1985-1992. *Neurology* 1994;44:1892-1900.

5. Gillespie SM, Chang Y, Leinp G, et al: Progressive multifocal leukoencephalopathy in persons infected with human immunodeficiency virus, San Francisco 1981-1989. *Ann Neurol* 1991;30:597-604.

6. von Einsiedel RW, Fife TD, Aksarmit AJ, et al: Progressive multifocal leukoencephalopathy in AIDS: A clinicopathologic study and review of the literature. *J Neurol* 1993;240:391-409.

7. Britton CB, Romagnoli M, Disi M, et al: Progressive multifocal leukoencephalopathy: disease progression, stabilization and response to intrathecal ARA-C in 26 patients. VII International Conference on AIDS/III STD World Congress. July, 1992, Amsterdam, The Netherlands 1:1512.

8. Holland NR, Power C, Mathews UP, et al: Cytomegalovirus encephalitis in acquired immunodeficiency syndrome. *Neurol* 1994;44:507-514.

9. Clifford DB, Butler RS, Mohammed S, et al: Use of polymerase chain reaction to demonstrate DNA in cerebrospinal fluid of patients with human immunodeficiency virus infection. *Neurol* 1993;43:75-79.

10. Brew BJ, Miller J: Human immunodeficiency virus type 1-related transient neurological defects. *Am J Med* 1996;101:257-261.

11. McArthur JC, Hoover DR, Bacellar H, et al: Dementia in AIDS patients. Incidence and risk factors. *Neurol* 1993;43:2245-2252.

12. Satz P, Morgenstein H, Miller EV, et al: Low education as a possible risk factor for cognitive abnormalities in HIV-1: findings from the MACS. *J Acquir Immune Defic Syndr* 1993;6:503-511.

13. Glass JD, Wesselingh SL, Selnes OA, et al: Clinical-neuropathologic correlation in HIV-associated dementia. *Neurol* 1993;43:2230-2237.

14. Brew BJ, Bhalla RB, Paul M, et al: Cerebrospinal fluid β_2-microglobulin in patients with AIDS dementia complex: an expanded series including response to zidovudine treatment. *AIDS* 1992;6:461-465.

Chapter 11

Neoplasia Related to HIV

The neoplastic conditions that the Centers for Disease Control and Prevention (CDC) includes in the definition of AIDS are Kaposi's sarcoma, non-Hodgkin's lymphoma (including B-cell lymphoma of the central nervous system), and cervical carcinoma.[1,2] Kaposi's sarcoma and non-Hodgkin's lymphoma were increasingly prevalent in immunodeficient patients even before the HIV-1 epidemic. Therefore, it is not surprising that they were recognized early as part of the syndrome and included in the CDC's first surveillance definition.[2] Cervical intraepithelial neoplasia and invasive cervical carcinoma were later found to be increasing in women infected with HIV-1 and were added to the surveillance definition most recently published by the CDC.[1] Other malignant conditions commonly reported in HIV-1 infected persons include Hodgkin's lymphoma; squamous cell carcinomas of the head, neck, and anus; melanoma; small cell carcinomas of the lung; testicular germ-cell tumors; and basal-cell carcinomas of the skin.[3] This chapter focuses on the three malignant conditions included in the current surveillance definition.

Kaposi's sarcoma (KS), endemic in central Africa but originally described among older men of Mediterranean origin, was recognized in the earliest cases of HIV-1 infection.

Formerly a rarely diagnosed condition, KS is now a common tumor managed in medical centers caring for HIV-1 infected persons. Kaposi's sarcoma was a common AIDS-defining condition in the United States when homosexual men were the predominant population subgroup with the syndrome. As the epidemic spread to injection drug users, to recipients of contaminated blood or blood products, and to women and children, KS became proportionally less common, as it rarely occurs in these populations. This epidemiologic evidence suggested to some clinicians that KS might be caused by a second, sexually transmitted agent or by an agent associated with the homosexual population.[4] Inhaled nitrite, used as a sexual stimulant by some homosexual men, was suggested as a possible link to development of KS in this HIV-1 infected group.[5] However, more recent studies have supported an infectious etiology. Using molecular techniques, Chang et al[6] detected DNA with homology to a herpesvirus in KS tissue. Later evidence suggested that the putative herpesvirus was also associated with a rare form of body cavity lymphoma. Extension of these studies documented that the KS herpesvirus, or herpesvirus type 8, was associated with African KS, the KS of older men, and the KS found in homosexual men not infected with HIV-1.[7,8]

The virus has recently been isolated and serologic techniques are now available that can detect the antibody before the development of KS in homosexual men.[9] A low level of endemic seropositivity has been documented in persons living in regions where the prevalence of KS has risen. The relationship of this herpesvirus to immunodeficiency and the pathogenetic mechanisms underlying development of KS have not yet been defined.

Other investigations have documented that KS lesions produce large amounts of cytokines that act in autocrine and paracrine fashions to enhance neoangiogenesis as well as spindle cell, fibroblast, and endothelial cell proliferation, all components of the tumor. Thus, cytokine dysregulation appears to be involved in the pathogenesis of KS.[10,11] Although some anecdotal reports have associated the use of antiherpes agents with a reduced preva-

Table 1: Staging of Kaposi's Sarcoma*

	Low Risk	High Risk
Tumor	localized to skin, oral cavity	tumor-associated edema, ulceration or viscera KS
Immune status	$CD4^+$ cells $> 200/mm^3$	$CD4^+$ cells $< 100/mm^3$
Clinical status	asymptomatic, Karnofsky status ≥ 70	major and minor HIV-1 related complications, fever, night sweats, diarrhea, weight loss, Karnofsky status ≤ 70

*Modified from Krown et al[12]

lence of KS, this benefit has not been definitely established. Therefore, the management of KS has been based on the chemotherapy of malignant disease.

Kaposi's sarcoma commonly involves the skin and may present as relatively insignificant ecchymotic-like lesions. But in HIV-1 infected persons, KS is unpredictable and can involve the pulmonary tract, gastrointestinal tract, or other internal organs. The oropharynx and the head and neck are common presenting sites of KS. Kaposi's sarcoma may be indolent, or explode and rapidly involve many sites. It can occur with $CD4^+$ lymphocyte counts that exceed $300/mm^3$, but in patients with advanced immunosuppression, KS is clearly more aggressive and can lead to death when it involves the viscera. A useful staging system has been proposed by Krown and colleagues (Table 1), based on the characteristics of the tumor, on the patient's immune status, and on presence or absence of systemic illness.[12]

Therapy is dictated by the stage of KS. Minimal disease often is not treated unless it is cosmetically disfiguring. In that case, radiation, intralesional injection of 0.01 mg of vincristine in 0.1 mL of sterile water, or cryotherapy are used.[13] A recent report suggested that intralesional injection of chorionic gonadotrophin leads to regression of KS lesions.[14] But it is not clear if this regression is the result of contaminant in commercial preparations or of the hormone. For widespread but slowly progressive disease in patients with more than $200/mm^3$ $CD4^+$ lymphocytes, antiretroviral therapy plus interferon-α, at dosages of less than 20 million U per day, has the advantage of combining the antiretroviral and antiproliferative activity of interferon with therapy that inhibits HIV-1 replication.[15,16] This therapy has been successful in stabilizing the condition.[15,16] When combined with interferon, zidovudine (Retrovir®) and other marrow-suppressive antiviral compounds often require the use of growth factors to prevent neutropenia.

For progressive widespread disease, more aggressive chemotherapy with doxorubicin (Adriamycin®), or with a combination of doxorubicin, bleomycin (Blenoxane®), and vincristine (Oncovin®) is used. Liposomal encapsulated doxorubicin and daunorubicin (Cerubidine®) are now available and response rates have been gratifying. Although associated with less systemic toxicity, these agents are myelosuppressive and they often require growth-factor therapy when administered.[3]

Non-Hodgkin's Lymphoma

The incidence of non-Hodgkin's lymphoma is significantly increased in all patients with immunosuppression and has been a significant problem for HIV-1 infected patients. It most commonly occurs in patients with far advanced disease and markedly reduces their survival.[17] These lymphomas were originally thought to be primarily intermediate or high-grade B-cell non-Hodgkin's tumors.

Although Epstein-Barr virus DNA sequences are commonly detected in the monoclonal B-cell tumors of the central nervous system, the peripheral lymphomas are more heterogeneous and often polyclonal. Chromosomal translocation similar to those found in Burkitt's lymphoma are found in a minority of tumors. As in KS, cytokine dysregulation appears to play a role in the pathogenesis of these lymphomas.[3]

In contrast to KS, which is primarily diagnosed in homosexual men, non-Hodgkin's lymphoma occurs in all HIV-1 infected persons. Extranodal disease is extremely common at diagnosis and frequently involves the gastrointestinal tract. Central nervous system (CNS) lymphoma presents with mental status changes, focal neurologic deficits, seizures, and headache. Central nervous system lymphoma can present with multiple lesions or, when using imaging techniques, as a single, discrete, hypodense, contrast-enhancing lesion. If a single lesion is found with computed tomography (CT) or magnetic resonance imaging (MRI), a biopsy is required. A biopsy is also necessary if multiple lesions develop and the patient does not have antibody to *Toxoplasma gondii*.[18]

Combination chemotherapy with methotrexate, bleomycin, cyclophosphamide, vincristine, and dexamethasone (mBACOD); with cyclophosphamide, doxorubicin, vincristine, and prednisone (CHOP); or with methotrexate, doxorubicin, cyclophosphamide, vincristine, prednisone, and bleomycin (MACOP-B) have all been used to treat HIV-1 related non-Hodgkin's lymphoma. Poor marrow reserves and HIV-1 induced immunosuppression have led to the use of less aggressive chemotherapeutic regimens that are associated with less toxicity, fewer opportunistic infections, and outcomes that equal those achieved with aggressive therapy even when combined with growth factor administration to prevent neutropenia.[13] Primary CNS lymphoma is usually treated with radiation. Despite good initial responses overall, mortality is high with a survival of less than 4 months for most patients.[19]

Cervical/Rectal Cancer

Cervical carcinoma in women and anal/rectal carcinoma in men and women with HIV-1 infection are associated with infection with oncogenic human papillomavirus (HPV), types 16, 18, and 31. Women infected with HIV-1 who are also infected with HPV have a much greater risk of having abnormal results of cytologic examinations than women who are not coinfected. The more advanced the HIV-1 infection, the more likely the cervical cytologic results will be abnormal. When invasive and preinvasive cervical neoplastic changes are present with HIV-1 infection, a greater risk exists for recurrence and perianal involvement.[20]

The association of HIV-1 and HPV with anal carcinoma in men is similar to cervical neoplasia in women.[21] Some clinicians have suggested (and studies to validate the proposal are underway) that homosexual men have routine Pap smears to screen for anal neoplasia. All HIV-1 infected women should have Pap smears of the cervix annually, preferably every 6 months in the first year after diagnosis of HIV-1 infection. Many authorities also advocate a baseline colposcopy. Treatment, if indicated, should be managed by a gynecologist familiar with caring for women infected with HIV-1.

References

1. Centers for Disease Control: Revised classification system for HIV infection and expanded surveillance definition for AIDS among adolescents and adults. *MMWR* 1992;41(RR-17).

2. Jaffe JW, Bregman DJ, Selik RM: Acquired immunodeficiency syndrome in the United States; the first 1,000 cases. *J Infect Dis* 1983;148:339-345.

3. Kaplan LD, Northfelt SW: Malignancies associated with AIDS. In: Sande MA, Volberding PA, eds. *The Medical Management of AIDS*. 4th ed. Philadelphia, WB Saunders, 1995.

4. Jacobson LP, Armenian HK: An integrated approach to the epidemiology of Kaposi's sarcoma. *Curr Opin Oncol* 1995;7:450-455.

5. Haverkos HW, Pinsky PF, Drotman DD, et al: Disease manifestation among homosexual men with acquired immunodeficiency syn-

drome: a possible role of nitrites in Kaposi's sarcoma. *Sex Transm Dis* 1985;12:203-208.

6. Chang Y, Cesamen E, Pessin MS, et al: Identification of herpesvirus-like DNA sequences in KS tissue from HIV-1 infected men. *Science* 1994;266:1565-1569.

7. Huang YQ, Li JJ, Kaplan MH, et al: Human herpesvirus-like nucleic acid in various forms of Kaposi's sarcoma. *Lancet* 1995; 345:759-761.

8. Dupin N, Grandadim M, Calvez V, et al: Herpesvirus-like DNA sequences in patients with Mediterranean Kaposi's sarcoma. *Lancet* 1995;345:761-762.

9. Gao SJ, Kingsley LA, Hoover DR, et al: Seroconversion to antibodies against Kaposi's sarcoma-associated herpesvirus-related latent nuclear antigens before development of Kaposi's sarcoma. *N Engl J Med* 1996;335:233-241.

10. Ensoli B, Nakamura S, Salahudden SZ, et al: AIDS-Kaposi's sarcoma-derived cells express cytokines with autocrine and paracrine growth effects. *Science* 1989;243:223-226.

11. Miles SA, Rezai AR, Salazar-Gonzalez JF, et al: AIDS Kaposi's sarcoma-derived cells produce and respond to interleukin 6. *Proc Natl Acad Sci U S A* 1990;83:4068-4072.

12. Krown S, Metroka C, Wernz J: Kaposi's sarcoma in the acquired immunodeficiency syndrome. A proposal for uniform evaluation, response and staging criteria. *J Clin Oncol* 1989;7:1201-1207.

13. Chak LY, Gill PS, Levine PM, et al: Radiation therapy for acquired-immunodeficiency syndrome-related Kaposi's sarcoma. *J Clin Oncol* 1988;6:863-867.

14. Gill PS, Lunardi-Iskandar Y, Louie S, et al: The effects of preparations of human chronic gonadotropin on AIDS-related Kaposi's sarcoma. *N Engl J Med* 1996;335:1261-1269.

15. Evans LM, Itri LM, Campion M, et al: Interferon-alpha 2a in treatment of acquired immunodeficiency syndrome-related Kaposi's sarcoma. *J Immunother* 1991;10:39-50.

16. Kovacs JA, Deyton L, Davey R, et al: Combined zidovudine and interferon-alpha therapy in patients with Kaposi's sarcoma and the acquired immunodeficiency syndrome. *Ann Intern Med* 1989;111:280-287.

17. Armenian HK, Hoover DR, Rubb S, et al: Risk factors for non-Hodgkin's lymphoma in acquired immunodeficiency syndrome. *Am J Epidemiol* 1996;143:374-379.

18. Rosenblum ML, Bredesen DE, Levy RM: Algorithms for the treatment of AIDS patients with neurological disease. In: Rosenblum ML, Levy RM, Bredesen DE, eds. *AIDS and the Nervous System*, New York, Raven Press, 1988.

19. Baumgartner J, Rachlin J, Beckstead J, et al: Primary central nervous system lymphomas: natural history and response to radiation therapy in 55 patients with acquired immunodeficiency syndrome. *J Neurosurg* 1990;73:206-211.

20. Maiman M, Fructer RG, Serur E, et al: Human immunodeficiency virus infection and cervical neoplasia. *Gynecol Oncol* 1990;38:377-382.

21. Palefsky JM, Gonzalez J, Greenblatt RM, et al: Anal intraepithelial neoplasia and anal papillomavirus infection among homosexual males with group IV HIV disease. *JAMA* 1990;263:2911-2916.

Index

NOTES

NOTES

NOTES